THE ULTIMATE

Herbal Compendium

A DESKTOP GUIDE FOR HERBAL PRESCRIBERS

by Kerry Bone

Associate Professor
School of Health
University of New England NSW Australia

PHYTOTHERAPY PRESS

Best wishes
Claudia

[signature] Kerry Bone

Columbus 2011

MW01077834

First Edition July 2007

Published by Phytotherapy Press,
PO Box 661, Warwick, Queensland 4370
Telephone +61 7 4661 9653

ISBN 978-0-646-47602-5

Design and layout by Sue Hamlet
Fledge Design Studio, Warwick, Queensland

Printed by Creed & Lang, Warwick,
Queensland

This book is written for professional
prescribing and should not be taken as a
guide to self treatment.

Table of Contents

Author's Preface

For some time now I have felt the need in my practice for an up-to-date, accurate and reliable ready reference. In a busy practice the time between taking a case and arriving at a final prescription can be relatively short. Decisions have to be made quickly, comprehensively and accurately, drawing on the best available information. Relying on memory is not always the best option and the currently available texts do not fully meet all the clinical requirements. I felt there was a role for a book that contained easily found information on a wide range of herbs and conditions, including doses for herbs in tablet form as well as the liquids.

This compendium has been developed with these requirements in mind. I have carefully researched, compiled and cross-referenced the available herbal information. But above all I was guided and informed by my clinical experience. As such, this compendium represents the distillation of more than 23 years of clinical practice.

A few key points are worthy of special mention. In order to make this book more compact and user-friendly, it is not referenced. However, all the sources used in compiling the information are listed in the bibliography section. If further detail is sought, then these sources can always be referred to. Also the book is intended as a quick reference for the younger herbal clinician or as a memory aid or prompt for the more experienced practitioner. Its contents are aimed to ensure that all valid herbal treatment options are considered. However, this compendium was never intended to replace good scholarship or adequate research into a case, and above all it should not replace the due consideration of the needs of the individual patient. Hence it can be regarded as a starting point or clinical tool that will lead to further ideas or insights as to how to treat a particular case. Alternatively, it can be used to check that a particular approach already in mind has merit, or to clarify the right dose for a particular herb and so on.

One of the most valuable features of this book is the comprehensive listings of herbs by their actions. I have long advocated that an appreciation of the herbal actions is a critical aspect of good herbal prescribing. Too often western herbalism is reduced to: "Which herbs are good for ....?" In reality, the key question is: "Which herbal actions are required for the treatment of this patient?" Hence when referring to the Therapeutic Index, where the herbs are listed according to medical conditions, the temptation to take this information at face value should be avoided. Instead the reader is encouraged to understand, by referring back to the Materia Medica section, why those herbs have been chosen for that particular disorder. This understanding is ultimately based on a well-considered knowledge of the herbs in terms of their clinically valid actions, together with an appreciation of what herbal actions are needed to treat that condition. Finally, to make the most of the information in this book it is important to be familiar with the How to Use section that follows this preface.

I hope that you can find a place for this herbal compendium on your consulting room desk.

A copy already sits on mine!

Kerry Bone

Warwick Australia 2007

Acknowledgements

Thanks to Amanda Williams and Jennifer Driscoll for their assistance in the conceptual development of this book.

Many thanks to my wife Patricia and to Vicki Matthews for their invaluable assistance with the development of the manuscript.

How to Use this Desktop Compendium

This compendium is divided into five main sections.

The Materia Medica section contains the essential prescribing information for around 190 herbs.

The second section (Actions Index) lists all these herbs in terms of their actions.

The third section (Therapeutic Index) details the herbs to be considered in the treatment of approximately 400 conditions.

The fourth section (Treatment Protocols) provides detailed example protocols for about 50 major conditions.

Finally, there is a classification of the herbs under their various contraindications and cautions, including important drug interactions as a separate listing.

Following this there are two appendices: Appendix 1 contains a glossary of all the herbal actions mentioned in this text and Appendix 2 gives the assumed tablet formulations that are used in the example protocols.

MATERIA MEDICA

Only the key prescribing information has been included in a summary format. Where appropriate, doses have been provided for both solid (tablet) and liquid forms of the herbal extract. The doses given are adult doses for the long-term administration of the herb. For children, the correct dose can be calculated according to their body weight. Take the weight of the child and divide by 60 (for kg) or 132 (for lbs) to find the fraction of the adult dose that is appropriate.

Doses are followed by the main actions. These actions have been carefully selected as representing the clinical activity of the herb. Often in herbal texts the actions assigned to a given herb are too many. This can leave the reader confused as to what are the key activities of a given herb that differentiate it from the others.

The indications listing is divided into two sections. The "Key Indications" are those that represent a consensus view on how the herb is best used clinically. The "Other Indications" are those that can be reasonably inferred from research, clinical experience or the known properties of the herb.

To make the Materia Medica more user-friendly, the indications are grouped as much as possible around themes. Sometimes various qualifiers are given in brackets. For example, the qualifier "acute doses" means that the long-term doses can be exceeded by a factor of 2 or 3 for short-term use, in the order of a few days or weeks. Where a qualifier, such as "acute doses" occurs at the end of an indications grouping and is preceded by the word "all", this means that the qualification applies to all the indications in that grouping. For an example, see the key indications for Bearberry. The qualifier "high doses" means that doses at the higher end of the given dosage range are appropriate.

The major safety issues section only lists those safety concerns that are of a high significance and relevance to clinical practice. For more detailed information on safety *The Essential Guide to Herbal Safety* is recommended (see the Bibliography).

Finally, key constituents are briefly listed, together with any significant quality or adulteration issues.

ACTIONS INDEX

The Actions Index has been drawn from the Materia Medica section and contains listings of herbs grouped by the actions in alphabetical order. A glossary at the end of the book provides definitions for these terms. Actions are the concepts that link the treatment goals or treatment framework to the choice of herbs. These are traditional herbal concepts, but scientific research also yields information about the actions of a herb. The stepwise process in linking treatment goals to choice of herbs for a prescription is then as follows.

1. Decide the treatment goals based on traditional herbal concepts, the orthodox medical understanding of the disorder and the patient's case.

2. Ensure that the goals are individualised to the requirements of the individual case.

3. Decide upon the immediate priorities of treatment.

4. On the basis of the immediate treatment goals, decide what actions are required.

5. Choose reliable herbs that have these actions, with as much overlap as possible. For example, if anti-inflammatory and spasmolytic actions are required for the gut, Chamomile can effectively cover both these requirements.

6. If a particular action needs to be reinforced, this can be achieved by choosing more than one herb with this action or by using a very effective herb in a higher dose.

7. Combine the herbs in a formula with appropriate doses. For a liquid formulation, do not choose too many herbs as this will compromise their individual doses in the formula and may lead to undefined interactions.

To facilitate this process, the herbal clinician needs a clear understanding of herbs in terms of their reliable, well-established actions. The provided reference list of herbs classified under each action is therefore a vital clinical resource.

THERAPEUTIC INDEX

The Therapeutic Index section contains herbs listed by indications. These lists were largely compiled from the Materia Medica section, but have been supplemented where relevant by the inclusion of additional herbs. Additional herbs were selected on the basis of a knowledge of the actions required for the appropriate treatment of each medical condition in question. The herbs are again listed in alphabetical order. Where there are many herbs listed for a particular condition, they are often divided into "Key" and "Other". This assignation of a key or supplementary role in a given medical condition largely follows the "Key" and "Other" classification in the Materia Medica section, but not necessarily.

A major feature of the Therapeutic Index is the extensive use of cross-referencing. A key aspect of this cross-referencing is that medical synonyms are cross-referenced as appropriate. For example "Gall bladder, infection" is cross-referenced to "Cholecystitis", so that the entry reads "Gall bladder, infection (see Cholecystitis)". But there is also extensive therapeutic cross-referencing, using the term "see also". Taking the example of blepharitis, this condition is typically linked to rosacea or chronic infection. Hence the heading for blepharitis reads "Blepharitis (see also Rosacea and Infection, chronic)". If the patient's blepharitis is linked to rosacea, then the herbs listed under both "Blepharitis" and "Rosacea" are relevant to the treatment. The final herb selection from these lists should then be determined by the individual case, the other additional actions required and the clinical reliability of the listed herbs. So if a gut antimicrobial action was also required for the patient with blepharitis, then Golden Seal would be chosen from the herbs listed under "Blepharitis", since it possesses the additional required action (gut antimicrobial) and is a clinically reliable herb. This example of how to approach the final selection of herbs can be usefully applied throughout the therapeutic section.

TREATMENT PROTOCOLS

Example treatment protocols are provided for the treatment of 50 common health problems. Both tablet and liquid protocols are given. Again, like the Therapeutic Index section, this information is best regarded as a guide, and should always be appropriately qualified and modified according to the individual patient and his or her unique needs. The tablet protocols provide examples of how this individualisation can be done.

For the tablet protocols, certain fixed combinations of herbs were assumed. Each combination is based on a therapeutic theme. Also some tablets have been assumed to contain just a single herb when these products are common in the marketplace. The example tablet formulations assumed for the protocols are provided in Appendix 2.

How to Use this Compendium

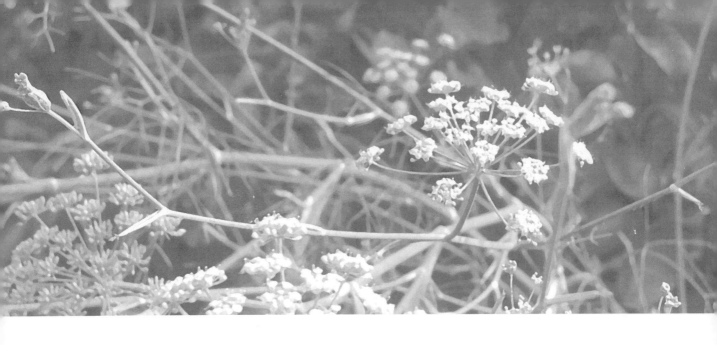

Materia Medica

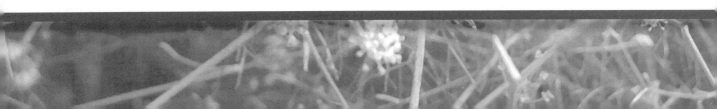

ADHATODA

Botanical Names(s)	Adhatoda vasica
Part Used	Leaf
Dose	20 to 30 mL/week (1:2 liquid) 1.5 to 2.3 g/day (tablet)
Main Actions	Expectorant, bronchospasmolytic, oxytocic
Key Indications	Asthma Chronic bronchitis Acute bronchitis (acute doses)
Other Indications	Gingivitis, bleeding gums (locally) Post-partum haemorrhage (acute doses)
Major Safety Issues	Contraindicated in pregnancy except at birth
Key Constituents	About 1% alkaloids including vasicine and vasicinone
Quality or Adulteration Issues	Leaf should contain adequate levels of key alkaloids

AGRIMONY

Botanical Names(s)	Agrimonia eupatoria
Part Used	Aerial parts
Dose	20 to 30 mL/week (1:2 liquid)
Main Actions	Mild astringent
Key Indications	Mild diarrhoea Haemorrhoids Urinary incontinence Venous insufficiency
Other Indications	Topically for haemorrhoids, venous insufficiency, dermatitis Cutaneous porphyria
Major Safety Issues	None known
Key Constituents	Tannins, flavonoids, triterpenic and phenolic acids

Quality or Adulteration Issues	No issues identified

ALBIZIA

Botanical Names(s)	Albizia lebbeck; Albizzia lebbeck
Part Used	Stem bark
Dose	25 to 60 mL/week (1:2 liquid) 2.4 to 4.0 g/day (tablet)
Main Actions	Antiallergic, hypocholesterolaemic
Key Indications	Hay fever Asthma Dermatitis (eczema) Urticaria
Other Indications	Hypercholesterolaemia (possible benefit)
Major Safety Issues	None known
Key Constituents	Not well defined. Saponins, tannins and flavonoids
Quality or Adulteration Issues	Important to ensure the correct species

ALFALFA

Botanical Names(s)	Medicago sativa
Part Used	Aerial parts
Dose	30 to 60 mL/week (1:2 liquid)
Main Actions	Oestrogen modulating, nutrient
Key Indications	Debility Menopausal symptoms
Major Safety Issues	Best avoided in oestrogen-sensitive breast cancer
Key Constituents	Isoflavones, vitamins, coumestrol and alkaloids asparagine and trigonelline

Quality or Adulteration Issues	No issues identified

ALOES RESIN

Botanical Names(s)	Aloe barbadensis; Aloe capensis
Part Used	Resin
Dose	10 to 30 mL/week (1:10 liquid)
Main Actions	Laxative
Key Indications	Constipation
Other Indications	Haemorrhoids (to soften the stool) Anal fissure (to soften the stool)
Major Safety Issues	Should only be used for short periods (8-10 days) Caution in pregnancy, lactation, irritable bowel syndrome and gastrointestinal inflammation Caution in children
Key Constituents	Anthraquinone glycosides including barbaloin
Quality or Adulteration Issues	Aloes resin should not be confused with the mucilage-containing Aloe vera juice or gel

ANDROGRAPHIS

Botanical Names(s)	Andrographis paniculata
Part Used	Aerial parts
Dose	20 to 40 mL/week (1:2 liquid) 4.0 to 6.0 g/day (tablet)
Main Actions	Immune enhancing, choleretic, hepatoprotective, anthelmintic
Key Indications	Acute infections: viral, bacterial or parasitic (all acute doses) Chronic infections Infection prevention Infective hepatitis (especially useful, acute doses)

	Intestinal worms (acute doses) Liver insufficiency, digestive weakness Acne
Other Indications	Flatulence Immune support in asthma
Major Safety Issues	Best avoided in the first trimester of pregnancy Use cautiously with immunosuppressive drugs
Key Constituents	Andrographolides including andrographolide itself
Quality or Adulteration Issues	Can be adulterated with other species and commercial extracts can be low in andrographolide

ANGELICA ROOT

Botanical Names(s)	Angelica archangelica
Part Used	Root
Dose	5 to 20 mL/week (1:2 liquid)
Main Actions	Aromatic digestive, carminative, diaphoretic, expectorant
Key Indications	Digestive weakness, flatulence Dyspepsia, anorexia Hypochlorhydria
Other Indications	Acute bronchitis, pleurisy Buerger's disease
Major Safety Issues	May cause photosensitivity, hence avoid prolonged exposure to sunlight. Caution in peptic ulcers and gastro-oesophageal reflux
Key Constituents	Furanocoumarins, essential oil and phenolic acids
Quality or Adulteration Issues	Other species of Angelica

ANISEED

Botanical Names(s)	Pimpinella anisum
Part Used	Fruit
Dose	20 to 40 mL/week (1:2 liquid) 350 to 700 mg essential oil/day
Main Actions	Expectorant, oestrogen modulating, galactagogue, spasmolytic, carminative, antimicrobial
Key Indications	Intestinal colic, flatulence, flatulent colic, infantile colic, dyspepsia Acute or chronic bronchitis, bronchial asthma Gastrointestinal candidiasis or parasites, to modify bowel flora
Other Indications	Difficult lactation Pertussis, spasmodic cough
Major Safety Issues	Caution in gastro-oesophageal reflux
Key Constituents	Essential oil (1.5 to 5%) containing mainly trans-anethole, fixed oil, flavonoids and phenylpropenyl esters
Quality or Adulteration Issues	Herb should contain at least 2% essential oil

ARNICA

Botanical Names(s)	Arnica montana, Arnica chamissonis subsp. foliosa
Part Used	Flower
Dose	Topical use only. Use diluted (2 to 3 times) 1:5 tincture or cream containing 2 to 5% herb equivalent
Main Actions	Topical actions: anti-inflammatory, antiecchymotic, analgesic
Key Indications	Topical use for: Osteoarthritis Bruises, sprains Varicose veins Venous insufficiency Myalgia
Other Indications	Topical use for: Furunculosis Inflamed insect bites
Major Safety Issues	Not for internal use
Key Constituents	Sesquiterpene lactones including helenalin, flavonoids, essential oil
Quality or Adulteration Issues	Often substituted with Mexican Arnica (Heterotheca inuloides)

ASTRAGALUS

Botanical Names(s)	Astragalus membranaceus
Part Used	Root
Dose	30 to 60 mL/week (1:2 liquid) 2.5 to 3.4 g/day (tablet)
Main Actions	Immune enhancing, tonic, adaptogen, cardiotonic, hypotensive, diuretic
Key Indications	Chronic infections Infection prevention (especially in depleted patients) Night sweats, chronic immune deficiency, poor immunity Debility, fatigue Leukopaenia Chronic fatigue syndrome, fibromyalgia, post-viral syndromes Mild congestive cardiac failure, bronchiectasis

	During chemotherapy or radiotherapy for cancer
Other Indications	Organ prolapse HIV/AIDS Angina pectoris
Major Safety Issues	Not advisable in acute infections. Use cautiously with immunosuppressive drugs
Key Constituents	Triterpenoid saponins (astragalosides), flavonoids, polysaccharides
Quality or Adulteration Issues	Can be substituted with other species of Astragalus

BACOPA

Botanical Names(s)	Bacopa monnieri; Bacopa monniera
Part Used	Aerial parts
Dose	35 to 90 mL/week (1:2 liquid) 7.5 to 10.0 g/day (tablet)
Main Actions	Cognition enhancing, nervine tonic, anxiolytic, mild anticonvulsant, thyroid stimulant
Key Indications	To improve memory (especially medium and long-term) To improve concentration or mental performance ADHD Alzheimer's disease
Other Indications	Insomnia, anxiety Epilepsy Cerebrovascular disease Hypothyroidism
Major Safety Issues	Saponins may cause or aggravate gastro-oesophageal reflux

Key Constituents	Dammarane-type saponins (loosely described as bacosides), flavonoids
Quality or Adulteration Issues	Centella asiatica has the same name in India (Brahmi) and is a common adulterant

BAICAL SKULLCAP

Botanical Names(s)	Scutellaria baicalensis
Part Used	Root
Dose	30 to 60 mL/week (1:2 liquid) 2.4 to 3.2 g/day (tablet)
Main Actions	Antiallergic, antioxidant, anti-inflammatory
Key Indications	Asthma, hay fever, dermatitis (eczema), urticaria Acute infections, especially respiratory and gastrointestinal (all acute doses) Hypertension
Other Indications	Diabetic neuropathy (to prevent) Restless foetus During chemotherapy
Major Safety Issues	Best avoided in the first trimester of pregnancy
Key Constituents	Flavones and flavone glycosides such as baicalin, baicalein and wogonin in high amounts
Quality or Adulteration Issues	The flavonoids can decompose over time

BAPTISIA

Botanical Names(s)	Baptisia tinctoria
Part Used	Root
Dose	15 to 40 mL/week (1:2 liquid)
Main Actions	Lymphatic, antipyretic, immune enhancing
Key Indications	Acute and chronic infections, especially respiratory

	Pneumonia, influenza, tonsillitis
	Enlarged lymph glands
Other Indications	Septic conditions, furunculosis
	Mouth ulcers, gingivitis
Major Safety Issues	None known
Key Constituents	Not well defined: cytisine (an alkaloid), coumarins, flavonoids, glycoproteins
Quality or Adulteration Issues	No issues identified

BARBERRY

Botanical Names(s)	Berberis vulgaris
Part Used	Root and/or stem bark
Dose	20 to 40 mL/week (1:2 liquid)
Main Actions	Antimicrobial, cholagogue, choleretic,antiemetic, bitter tonic, antiparasitic
Key Indications	Digestive liver insufficiency, dyspepsia
	Gall stones, cholecystitis, gall bladder dysfunction
	Peptic ulcer, gastritis (involving Helicobacter)
	Acute gastrointestinal infection with diarrhoea (non-viral)
	Hypertyraminaemia
Other Indications	Bowel flora, to modify
	Nausea
	Acne (topically)
	Thrombocytopaenia
Major Safety Issues	Best avoided during pregnancy and lactation
Key Constituents	Protoberberine alkaloids including berberine, jatrorrhizine and palmatine
Quality or Adulteration Issues	Other species of Berberis can be encountered as adulterants

BAYBERRY

Botanical Names(s)	Myrica cerifera
Part Used	Root bark
Dose	15 to 40 mL/week (1:2 liquid)
Main Actions	Astringent, circulatory stimulant, mild diaphoretic, mild choleretic
Key Indications	Diarrhoea
	Common cold
Other Indications	Leucorrhoea (as a douche)
	Sore throat (as a gargle)
Major Safety Issues	Take away from mineral supplements, thiamine or alkaloids
Key Constituents	Not well defined. Triterpenes including myricadiol, flavonoids including myricitrin
Quality or Adulteration Issues	No issues identified

BEARBERRY

Botanical Names(s)	Arctostaphylos uva-ursi
Part Used	Leaf
Dose	30 to 60 mL/week (1:2 liquid)
	1.5 to 2.0 g/day (tablet)
Main Actions	Urinary antiseptic, astringent, anti-inflammatory
Key Indications	Cystitis, urethritis, dysuria (all acute doses)
	Recurrent cystitis
Other Indications	Acute prostatitis (acute doses)
	Kidney and bladder stones
	Topically for melasma
Major Safety Issues	Contraindicated in pregnancy, lactation, kidney disease and children under 12 years. Take away from mineral supplements, thiamine or alkaloids

Key Constituents	Hydroquinone glycosides (including arbutin and methylarbutin), tannins
Quality or Adulteration Issues	Leaf containing less than 6% arbutin should be considered to be adulterated

BETH ROOT

Botanical Names(s)	Trillium erectum; Trillium pendulum
Part Used	Root
Dose	10 to 30 mL/week (1:2 liquid)
Main Actions	Antihaemorrhagic, astringent, mild expectorant, uterine tonic
Key Indications	Menorrhagia, metrorrhagia Post-partum haemorrhage Dysfunctional uterine bleeding
Other Indications	Leucorrhoea (as a douche)
Major Safety Issues	Saponins may cause or aggravate gastro-oesophageal reflux
Key Constituents	Not well defined. Saponins, fixed oil and tannins
Quality or Adulteration Issues	Important to ensure the correct species

BILBERRY

Botanical Names(s)	Vaccinium myrtillus
Part Used	Fruit
Dose	20 to 40 mL/week (1:1 liquid) 18 to 24 g/day (fresh weight, tablet)
Main Actions	Vasoprotective, antioedema, antioxidant, anti-inflammatory
Key Indications	Diabetic or hypertensive retinopathy Macular degeneration Eyestrain, night blindness, glaucoma Capillary fragility, bleeding gums

	Haemorrhoids, varicose veins, venous insufficiency (especially during pregnancy) To promote healing (especially after surgery)
Other Indications	Spasmodic dysmenorrhoea Spider veins Slowing of mental ageing
Major Safety Issues	None expected at recommended doses
Key Constituents	Anthocyanins, flavonoids, procyanidins
Quality or Adulteration Issues	Other species of Vaccinium have been noted as adulterants. Commercial extracts may be adulterated with artificial colouring agents

BLACK COHOSH

Botanical Names(s)	Cimicifuga racemosa; Actea racemosa
Part Used	Root and rhizome
Dose	10 to 20 mL/week (1:2 liquid) 300 to 400 mg/day (tablet)
Main Actions	Oestrogen modulating, uterine tonic, spasmolytic, antirheumatic
Key Indications	Menopausal symptoms Spasmodic dysmenorrhoea, premenstrual syndrome Osteoarthritis (especially small joint), rheumatoid arthritis To prepare for labour (in late pregnancy)
Other Indications	Myalgia Tinnitus
Major Safety Issues	Contraindicated during pregnancy (except in the last few weeks to assist with birth). Controversial in breast cancer
Key Constituents	Triterpenoid saponins (including actein and cimicifugoside), resin, caffeic and isoferulic acids

Quality or Adulteration Issues	Other species of Cimicifuga and Actea are known adulterants

BLACK HAW

Botanical Names(s)	Viburnum prunifolium
Part Used	Bark
Dose	10 to 30 mL/week (1:2 liquid)
Main Actions	Uterine spasmolytic, hypotensive, bronchospasmolytic, antiasthmatic, astringent
Key Indications	Spasmodic dysmenorrhoea (acute doses) Miscarriage, threatened or repeated
Other Indications	Post-partum haemorrhage Asthma
Major Safety Issues	None known
Key Constituents	Coumarins (scopoletin), flavonoids (amentoflavone), iridoid glycosides, tannins and triterpenes
Quality or Adulteration Issues	Several species including Acer spicatum are known adulterants

BLACK WALNUT

Botanical Names(s)	Juglans nigra
Part Used	Green hulls
Dose	10 to 40 mL/week (1:10 liquid)
Main Actions	Anthelmintic, depurative
Key Indications	Intestinal worms (pin worms, round worms etc)
Other Indications	Chronic skin disorders
Major Safety Issues	None known
Key Constituents	Naphthoquinones including juglone and plumbagin

Quality or Adulteration Issues	Important to use the green hulls

BLADDERWRACK

Botanical Names(s)	Fucus vesiculosis
Part Used	Thallus (plant body)
Dose	30 to 60 mL/week (1:1 liquid) 2 to 4 g/day (tablet)
Main Actions	Antiobesity, thyroid stimulant
Key Indications	Hypothyroidism, subclinical or clinical obesity (associated with poor thyroid activity)
Other Indications	Osteoarthritis (in association with obesity)
Major Safety Issues	Contraindicated in hyperthyroidism. Caution during pregnancy and lactation
Key Constituents	Iodine, more than half of which is organically bound to proteins, amino acids, polysaccharides
Quality or Adulteration Issues	Often adulterated with kelp (Laminaria species)

BLUE COHOSH

Botanical Names(s)	Caulophyllum thalictroides
Part Used	Root
Dose	10 to 20 mL/week (1:2 liquid)
Main Actions	Spasmolytic, uterine and ovarian tonic, emmenagogue, oxytocic
Key Indications	To assist with labour (in late pregnancy) Spasmodic dysmenorrhoea Ovarian pain
Other Indications	Uterine prolapse Secondary amenorrhoea Endometriosis

Major Safety Issues	Contraindicated in early pregnancy and lactation. Use in late pregnancy should only be undertaken by experienced clinicians
Key Constituents	Quinolizidine alkaloids, saponins
Quality or Adulteration Issues	No adulterants reported

BLUE FLAG

Botanical Names(s)	Iris versicolor; Iris caroliniana
Part Used	Rhizome
Dose	20 to 40 mL/week (1:2 liquid)
Main Actions	Depurative, mild laxative, lymphatic, cholagogue
Key Indications	Chronic skin disorders including dermatitis (eczema), acne, psoriasis, rosacea
	Digestive liver insufficiency and associated symptoms such as nausea, constipation and headache
	Enlarged lymph glands
Other Indications	Splenic enlargement
	To assist with weight loss
Major Safety Issues	No major issues noted
Key Constituents	Not well defined. Triterpenoids (iriversical), essential oil, resin
Quality or Adulteration Issues	Adulteration by other species of Iris is common

BONESET

Botanical Names(s)	Eupatorium perfoliatum
Part Used	Aerial parts
Dose	10 to 30 mL/week (1:2 liquid)
Main Actions	Diaphoretic
Key Indications	Influenza marked by severe myalgia ("breakbone fever") (acute doses)
Other Indications	Nasopharyngeal catarrh
Major Safety Issues	None known
Key Constituents	Sesquiterpene lactones, essential oil
Quality or Adulteration Issues	Other species of Eupatorium can be adulterants

BOSWELLIA

Botanical Names(s)	Boswellia serrata
Part Used	Oleogum resin
Dose	3.6 to 4.8 g/day (tablet)
Main Actions	Anti-inflammatory, antiarthritic, antitumour
Key Indications	Rheumatoid arthritis, osteoarthritis
	Crohn's disease, ulcerative colitis
	Asthma
	Oedema due to malignant brain tumours
Other Indications	Disorders characterised by elevated leukotrienes and cytokines such as cystic fibrosis, psoriasis, lupus, gout, urticaria, multiple sclerosis, hay fever
	Adjunct therapy in cancer
Major Safety Issues	No major problems identified
Key Constituents	Pentacyclic triterpene acids (boswellic acids), essential oil, terpenols, uronic acids and sterols
Quality or Adulteration Issues	Important to use extracts standardised for boswellic acids by HPLC

BUCHU

Botanical Names(s)	Barosma betulina; Agathosma betulina
Part Used	Leaf
Dose	15 to 30 mL/week (1:2 liquid) 36 to 48 mg/day (essential oil)
Main Actions	Urinary antiseptic, mild diuretic
Key Indications	Cystitis, urethritis, dysuria (all acute doses) Recurrent cystitis
Other Indications	Acute prostatitis (acute doses) Chronic prostatitis
Major Safety Issues	No major issues if the correct species is used
Key Constituents	Essential oil (including diosphenols and sulphur containing monoterpenes which give the characteristic odour), flavonoids (diosmin, rutin)
Quality or Adulteration Issues	Often substituted with other species of Agathosma which can create safety concerns

BUGLEWEED

Botanical Names(s)	Lycopus virginicus; Lycopus europaeus
Part Used	Aerial parts
Dose	15 to 40 mL/week (1:2 liquid)
Main Actions	Antithyroid, mild sedative
Key Indications	Hyperthyroidism and associated symptoms
Major Safety Issues	Contraindicated in hypothyroidism, pregnancy and lactation
Key Constituents	Phenolic acids and flavonoids
Quality or Adulteration Issues	Leonurus marrubiastrum may be mistaken for L. europaeus

BUPLEURUM

Botanical Names(s)	Bupleurum falcatum
Part Used	Root
Dose	25 to 60 mL/week (1:2 liquid) 1.2 to 2.8 g/day (tablet)
Main Actions	Anti-inflammatory, hepatoprotective, antitussive, diaphoretic
Key Indications	Autoimmune disease (especially involving the liver or kidneys) Hepatitis, liver damage, nausea Poor digestive liver function
Other Indications	Influenza, common cold Chronic cough Uterine prolapse (combined with Astragalus)
Major Safety Issues	Saponins may cause or aggravate gastro-oesophageal reflux
Key Constituents	Triterpenoid saponins (saikosaponins), phytosterols, polysaccharides (bupleurans)
Quality or Adulteration Issues	Other species of Bupleurum can be adulterants which can give rise to toxicity concerns

BURDOCK

Botanical Names(s)	Arctium lappa; Arctium majus
Part Used	Root
Dose	10 to 25 mL/week (1:2 liquid) 0.9 to 1.2 g/day (tablet)
Main Actions	Depurative, diuretic depurative
Key Indications	Chronic skin disorders including dermatitis (eczema), acne, psoriasis, rosacea Furunculosis
Other Indications	Gout, rheumatism, rheumatoid arthritis
Major Safety Issues	No major issues identified

Key Constituents	Essential oil, phenolic acids, sesquiterpene lactones, acetylenic compounds including nine containing sulphur, inulin
Quality or Adulteration Issues	Can be confused with other plants during wild harvesting, including Belladonna

BUTCHER'S BROOM

Botanical Names(s)	Ruscus aculeatus
Part Used	Root and rhizome
Dose	25 to 50 mL/week (1:2 liquid) 1.6 to 2.4 g/day (tablet)
Main Actions	Venotonic, anti-inflammatory, antioedema
Key Indications	Venous insufficiency Varicose veins, haemorrhoids Varicose ulcer Lymphoedema Premenstrual syndrome Deep vein thrombosis (to reduce risk)
Other Indications	Restless legs syndrome, leg cramps, night cramps Spider veins, capillary fragility, bruises, easy bruising
Major Safety Issues	Saponins may cause or aggravate gastro-oesophageal reflux
Key Constituents	Steroidal saponins (aglycones ruscogenin and neoruscogenin)
Quality or Adulteration Issues	No adulterants known

BUTTERNUT

Botanical Names(s)	Juglans cinerea
Part Used	Bark
Dose	25 to 50 mL/week (1:2 liquid)
Main Actions	Mild laxative, cholagogue, depurative
Key Indications	Constipation Poor digestive liver function
Other Indications	Exudative skin eruptions (dermatitis etc)
Major Safety Issues	None known
Key Constituents	Not well defined. Naphthoquinones (juglone), juglandic acid, essential oil, tannins
Quality or Adulteration Issues	No issues identified

CALENDULA

Botanical Names(s)	Calendula officinalis
Part Used	Flower
Dose	10 to 30 mL/week (1:2 liquid)
Main Actions	Vulnerary, lymphatic, anti-inflammatory, styptic (haemostatic), antimicrobial, antiviral (topically), antifungal (topically)
Key Indications	Internal treatment for: Peptic ulcers Enlarged lymph glands Acne, sebaceous cysts Spasmodic dysmenorrhoea Topical treatment for: Mouth ulcers, herpes simplex lesions Acne, dermatitis (eczema) Wounds, ulcers, varicose ulcer, bed sores Minor burns, inflamed skin, nappy rash Haemorrhoids, varicose veins Insect bites
Major Safety Issues	Contraindicated in known allergy to Calendula
Key Constituents	Triterpenoid saponins, triterpene alcohols and their monoesters, flavonoids, carotenoids, phenolic acids, coumarins and essential oil

Quality or Adulteration Issues	Adulteration is uncommon

CALIFORNIA POPPY

Botanical Names(s)	Eschscholtzia californica
Part Used	Aerial parts
Dose	20 to 40 mL/week (1:2 liquid)
Main Actions	Anxiolytic, mild sedative, analgesic, hypnotic
Key Indications	Pain management for nerve-generated pain (acute doses as required)
	Neuralgia, sciatica, trigeminal neuralgia, toothache, tension headache (all acute doses as required)
	Insomnia
	Anxiety, emotional stress
Other Indications	Panic attacks (acute doses)
Major Safety Issues	No major issues identified
Key Constituents	Isoquinoline alkaloids including californidine and eschscholtzine, some protopine alkaloids
Quality or Adulteration Issues	No adulterants known

CASCARA

Botanical Names(s)	Rhamnus purshiana
Part Used	Bark
Dose	20 to 55 mL/week (1:2 liquid)
	1 to 3 g/day (tablet)
Main Actions	Laxative
Key Indications	Constipation
	Haemorrhoids or anal fissure (to soften the stool, cathartic doses to be avoided)
Other Indications	Tension headache (linked to constipation)

Major Safety Issues	For short-term use only. Caution in pregnancy, lactation, irritable bowel syndrome and gastrointestinal inflammation. Caution in children. Contraindicated in diarrhoea or with digoxin
Key Constituents	Anthraquinone glycosides
Quality or Adulteration Issues	Can be adulterated with the barks of other Rhamnus species

CAT'S CLAW

Botanical Names(s)	Uncaria tomentosa
Part Used	Stem bark
Dose	30 to 75 mL/week (1:2 liquid)
	4.5 to 6.0 g/day (tablet)
Main Actions	Immune enhancing, anti-inflammatory, antioxidant
Key Indications	Poor immunity, tendency to infections
	Convalescence, debility, chronic immune deficiency
	HIV/AIDS
	Adjunct therapy in cancer
	Rheumatoid arthritis, osteoarthritis
Other Indications	Chronic fatigue syndrome, fibromyalgia
	Autoimmune disease
	Immune support in asthma or Lyme disease
Major Safety Issues	Contraindicated in pregnancy. Use cautiously with immunosuppressive drugs
Key Constituents	Pentacyclic and tetracyclic oxindole alkaloids (POA and TOA)
Quality or Adulteration Issues	Important to use a chemotype with predominantly POA content

CAYENNE

Botanical Names(s)	Capsicum annuum
Part Used	Fruit
Dose	0.5 to 3 mL/week (1:3 liquid)
Main Actions	Pungent, counterirritant, carminative, circulatory and metabolic stimulant, spasmolytic, diaphoretic
Key Indications	Impaired peripheral circulation, chilblains, intermittent claudication
	Hypochlorhydria, digestive weakness, flatulent colic
	Acute infections and fever
	To assist weight loss
	Topically for osteoarthritis, myalgia, rheumatoid arthritis, diabetic neuropathy, post-herpetic and other neuralgias, laryngitis, pharyngitis
Other Indications	Angina pectoris
	Raynaud's syndrome
Major Safety Issues	Caution in peptic ulcers and topical application to damaged skin. Compliance can be a problem. May cause gastro-oesophageal reflux
Key Constituents	Capsaicinoids, carotenoids, flavonoids and phenolic acids
Quality or Adulteration Issues	No issues identified

CELERY SEED

Botanical Names(s)	Apium graveolens
Part Used	Fruit
Dose	30 to 60 mL/week (1:2 liquid)
	3 to 4 g/day (tablet
Main Actions	Anti-inflammatory, antirheumatic, mild diuretic, diuretic depurative
Key Indications	Osteoarthritis, rheumatoid arthritis
	Gout, rheumatism
Major Safety Issues	Caution in kidney disorders
Key Constituents	Essential oil rich in phthalides (3-n-butyl phthalide, sedanenolide), flavonoids, coumarins and furanocoumarins
Quality or Adulteration Issues	Preparations rich in the phthalides will give the best therapeutic results

CHAMOMILE

Botanical Names(s)	Matricaria recutita; Chamomilla recutita
Part Used	Flower
Dose	20 to 40 mL/week (1:2 liquid)
	0.9 to 1.8 g/day (tablet)
	15 to 20 mg/day (essential oil)
Main Actions	Anti-inflammatory, spasmolytic, carminative, mild sedative, antiulcer, vulnerary, diaphoretic
Key Indications	Irritable bowel syndrome, food sensitivities
	Flatulent colic, flatulence, gastrointestinal tract colic and inflammation, diarrhoea
	Teething and infantile colic
	Gastritis, peptic ulcers, gastro-oesophageal reflux
	Topically for dermatitis, mouth ulcers, wounds
Other Indications	Travel sickness
	Restlessness, anxiety, insomnia, nervous dyspepsia
Major Safety Issues	Avoid in known allergy
Key Constituents	Essential oil (containing dicycloethers, bisabolol oxides and preferably bisabolol), matricine, flavonoids, coumarins

Quality or Adulteration Issues	Preparations rich in bisabolol will give the best therapeutic results

CHAPARRAL

Botanical Names(s)	Larrea tridentata
Part Used	Leaf
Dose	10 to 25 mL/week (1:2 liquid)
Main Actions	Depurative, antioxidant, antitumour
Key Indications	Adjunct therapy in cancer
Major Safety Issues	Use of this herb has been implicated in hepatotoxic reactions
Key Constituents	Resin containing lignans, principally nordihydroguaiaretic acid
Quality or Adulteration Issues	Other species of Larrea are known adulterants

CHASTE TREE

Botanical Names(s)	Vitex agnus-castus
Part Used	Fruit
Dose	5 to 40 mL/week (1:2 liquid) 0.25 to 3 g/day (tablet)
Main Actions	Prolactin inhibitor, dopaminergic agonist, indirectly progesterogenic, galactagogue
Key Indications	Premenstrual syndrome, especially with mastalgia Latent hyperprolactinaemia, erratic ovulation Acne (male and female) Relative oestrogen excess, polycystic ovary syndrome, cystic hyperplasia of the endometrium Uterine fibroids, endometriosis (higher doses) Oligomenorrhoea, polymenorrhoea, dysfunctional uterine bleeding, menorrhagia, metrorrhagia Amenorrhoea (to enhance fertility) Benign breast growths, ovarian cyst (follicular), painful ovulation Sleep maintenance insomnia Excessive libido in men (higher doses)
Other Indications	For premenstrual-like symptoms in association with menopause Post-natal depression Difficult lactation (now controversial) Threatened miscarriage
Major Safety Issues	Best not taken in conjunction with progestogenic drugs, the contraceptive pill or hormone replacement therapy. May aggravate pure spasmodic dysmenorrhoea not associated with premenstrual syndrome
Key Constituents	Diterpenes (including rotundifuran, vitexilactone), iridoid glycosides (agnuside, aucubin), flavonoids (casticin), essential oil
Quality or Adulteration Issues	Common adulterants of V. agnus-castus are V. negundo, V. rotundifolia and V. trifolia, which are Asiatic species used in Chinese or Ayurvedic medicine

CHEN PI

Botanical Names(s)	Citrus reticulata
Part Used	Fruit peel
Dose	25 to 50 mL/week (1:2 liquid) 1.5 to 2.0 g/day (tablet)
Main Actions	Carminative, aromatic digestive, expectorant
Key Indications	Digestive weakness, dyspepsia Anorexia

	Intestinal colic, abdominal bloating, flatulent colic
	Nausea, diarrhoea
	Food allergies/sensitivities
Major Safety Issues	None known
Key Constituents	Flavonoids (hesperidin), essential oil (limonene)
Quality or Adulteration Issues	No issues identified

CHICKWEED

Botanical Names(s)	Stellaria media
Part Used	Aerial parts
Dose	20 to 40 mL/week (1:2 liquid)
Main Actions	Demulcent, astringent, refrigerant, antiulcer (peptic)
Key Indications	Peptic ulcer
	Topically for dermatitis (eczema), psoriasis, other chronic skin disorders, wounds, insect bites and burns
Major Safety Issues	Avoid in known allergy (either topical or internal)
Key Constituents	Not well defined. Flavonoids, phenolic acids, triterpenoid saponins, phytosterols
Quality or Adulteration Issues	No adulterants known

CINNAMON, CASSIA OR CHINESE

Botanical Names(s)	Cinnamomum cassia, Cinnamomum aromatica
Part Used	Stem bark
Dose	10 to 30 mL/week (1:2 liquid)

Main Actions	Antidiabetic, carminative, stomachic, spasmolytic, mild astringent, aromatic digestive
Key Indications	Diabetes, metabolic syndrome X, insulin resistance (all higher doses)
	Flatulent colic, dyspepsia, digestive weakness
	Anorexia, nausea, diarrhoea
Other Indications	Common cold
Major Safety Issues	Caution in pregnancy and gastro-oesophageal reflux. Caution with patients on antidiabetic drugs. Take away from mineral supplements, thiamine or alkaloids
Key Constituents	Essential oil (high in cinnamaldehyde), coumarin, oxygenated diterpenes, proanthocyanidins
Quality or Adulteration Issues	No issues identified

CLIVERS

Botanical Names(s)	Galium aparine
Part Used	Aerial parts
Dose	25 to 50 mL/week (1:2 liquid)
	1.0 to 2.0 g/day (tablet)
Main Actions	Depurative, lymphatic, diuretic depurative
Key Indications	Chronic skin disorders including dermatitis (eczema), acne, psoriasis, rosacea
	Enlarged or inflamed lymph glands
Other Indications	Kidney stones, dysuria
Major Safety Issues	None required on current evidence
Key Constituents	Iridoid glycosides (monotropein), scopoletin, phenolic acids and flavonoids
Quality or Adulteration Issues	No adulterants known

CLOVES

Botanical Names(s)	Syzygium aromaticum; Eugenia caryophyllus
Part Used	Flower bud
Dose	10 to 25 mL/week (1:2 liquid) 60 to 120 mg/day (essential oil)
Main Actions	Anthelmintic, carminative, aromatic digestive, spasmolytic, cholagogue, antimicrobial, analgesic
Key Indications	Intestinal worms Flatulence, flatulent colic with abdominal bloating Nausea, dyspepsia Topically for toothache, pharyngitis, laryngitis, halitosis, to prevent dental caries
Major Safety Issues	Caution in gastro-oesophageal reflux
Key Constituents	Essential oil (high in eugenol), flavonoids, chromones, phenolic acids
Quality or Adulteration Issues	No issues identified

CODONOPSIS

Botanical Names(s)	Codonopsis pilosula
Part Used	Root
Dose	30 to 60 mL/week (1:2 liquid)
Main Actions	Tonic
Key Indications	Anaemia due to deficient red blood cell production Fatigue, anorexia, debility, convalescence
Other Indications	Adjunct therapy in cancer Chronic fatigue syndrome, fibromyalgia
Major Safety Issues	None known
Key Constituents	Not well defined. Sterols, triterpenes, essential oil and phenylpropanoid glycosides (tangshenosides)
Quality or Adulteration Issues	Campanumoea javania and Platycodon grandiflorus are known adulterants

COLEUS

Botanical Names(s)	Coleus forskohlii
Part Used	Root
Dose	40 to 90 mL/week (1:1 liquid) 7.5 to 11.0 g/day (tablet)
Main Actions	Hypotensive, antiplatelet, bronchospasmolytic, spasmolytic, cardiotonic, digestive stimulant, aromatic digestive, antiobesity
Key Indications	To assist with weight loss, metabolic syndrome X Hypertension, mild congestive cardiac failure, to prevent heart attacks (antiplatelet action) Asthma, chronic bronchitis, emphysema Hypothyroidism Digestive weakness, hypochlorhydria Psoriasis
Other Indications	Alcohol-free preparation topically for glaucoma Osteopaenia
Major Safety Issues	Caution in patients taking prescribed medication, especially hypotensive and antiplatelet drugs Contraindicated in hypotension and peptic ulcer
Key Constituents	Labdane diterpenes (including forskolin), essential oil
Quality or Adulteration Issues	Important to use extracts with sufficient quantity of forskolin

COMFREY

Botanical Names(s)	Symphytum officinale
Part Used	Leaf
Dose	Cream or ointment containing 10 to 30%
Main Actions	Anti-inflammatory, vulnerary, demulcent
Key Indications	Topical use for:
	Wounds, ulcers, insect bite
	Dermatitis (eczema), psoriasis
	Fractures, sprains
	Osteoarthritis, myalgia
Major Safety Issues	For topical use only
Key Constituents	Allantoin, mucilage, phenolic acids, pyrrolizidine alkaloids
Quality or Adulteration Issues	Digitalis is recorded as an accidental adulterant

CORN SILK

Botanical Names(s)	Zea mays
Part Used	Style and stigma
Dose	15 to 40 mL/week (1:1 liquid)
Main Actions	Urinary demulcent, antilithic, mild diuretic
Key Indications	Cystitis, urethritis, dysuria (all acute doses)
	Acute prostatitis (acute doses), chronic prostatitis
Other Indications	Enuresis
	Kidney stones
Major Safety Issues	None known
Key Constituents	Flavonoids (maysin), mucilage, tannins, essential oil, potassium
Quality or Adulteration Issues	No issues identified

CORYDALIS

Botanical Names(s)	Corydalis ambigua
Part Used	Tuber
Dose	25 to 60 mL/week (1:2 liquid) 1.8 to 3.6 g/day (tablet)
Main Actions	Mild sedative, hypnotic, analgesic, antiarrhythmic, spasmolytic
Key Indications	Pain management, especially for visceral pain
	Irritable bowel syndrome, spasmodic or congestive dysmenorrhoea, tension headache
	Insomnia, anxiety, emotional stress
	Cardiac arrhythmias, palpitations
Other Indications	BPH or chronic prostatitis as a spasmolytic
Major Safety Issues	Contraindicated during pregnancy
Key Constituents	Alkaloids including tetrahydropalmatine and corydalis L
Quality or Adulteration Issues	No issues identified

COUCH GRASS

Botanical Names(s)	Elymus repens; Agropyron repens
Part Used	Rhizome
Dose	20 to 40 mL/week (1:1 liquid)
Main Actions	Urinary demulcent, mild diuretic
Key Indications	Cystitis, urethritis, dysuria (all acute doses)
	Acute prostatitis (acute doses), chronic prostatitis
Other Indications	Kidney stones
Major Safety Issues	None known
Key Constituents	Not well defined. Polysaccharides (triticin), sugar alcohols, possibly saponins

Quality or Adulteration Issues	The principal adulterant is the rhizome of Cynodon dactylon. Imperata cylindrica and Carex spp. have also been noted as adulterants

CRAMP BARK

Botanical Names(s)	Viburnum opulus
Part Used	Bark
Dose	15 to 30 mL/week (1:2 liquid) 1.6 to 3.2 g/day (tablet)
Main Actions	Spasmolytic, hypotensive, peripheral vasodilator, mild sedative, astringent
Key Indications	Spasmodic dysmenorrhoea (acute doses), endometriosis Miscarriage (threatened or repeated) Hypertension To prepare for labour (in late pregnancy)
Other Indications	Irritable bowel syndrome, tension headache BPH or chronic prostatitis as a spasmolytic
Major Safety Issues	No major issues identified
Key Constituents	Not well defined. Catechin, epicatechin, coumarins (scopoletin, scopolin)
Quality or Adulteration Issues	Adulterants include Acer spicatum and other Viburnum species

CRANBERRY

Botanical Names(s)	Vaccinium macrocarpon
Part Used	Fruit
Dose	10 to 20 g/day (fresh weight, tablet)
Main Actions	Astringent, bacteriostatic
Key Indications	Cystitis (acute doses) Best for recurrent cystitis
Other Indications	Peptic ulcer (involving Helicobacter)
Major Safety Issues	Caution in patients taking warfarin and for oxalate kidney stones
Key Constituents	Procyanidins, catechin, epicatechin, anthocyanins
Quality or Adulteration Issues	Adulteration is unlikely

CRANESBILL

Botanical Names(s)	Geranium maculatum
Part Used	Root
Dose	15 to 35 mL/week (1:2 liquid)
Main Actions	Astringent, antidiarrhoeal, antihaemorrhagic, vulnerary, styptic
Key Indications	Diarrhoea, gastrointestinal bleeding Menorrhagia, metrorrhagia Topically for leucorrhoea, bleeding gums, pharyngitis, wounds, bleeding skin
Major Safety Issues	Long term use is best avoided due to the tannin content. Take away from mineral supplements, thiamine or alkaloids
Key Constituents	Hydrolysable tannins (up to 30%) including geraniin
Quality or Adulteration Issues	No issues identified

CRATAEVA

Botanical Names(s)	Crataeva nurvala
Part Used	Bark
Dose	40 to 100 mL/week (1:2 liquid) 3 to 6 g/day (tablet)
Main Actions	Antilithic, bladder tonic, anti-inflammatory

Key Indications	Cystitis, urethritis (all acute doses)
	Recurrent cystitis
	Kidney or bladder stones
	Hypotonic or atonic bladder, including for BPH
Other Indications	Incontinence, enuresis
Major Safety Issues	None known
Key Constituents	Sterols (lupeol), flavonoids, glucosinolates (glucocapparin)
Quality or Adulteration Issues	No issues identified

DAMIANA

Botanical Names(s)	Turnera diffusa; Turnera aphrodisiaca
Part Used	Leaf
Dose	20 to 40 mL/week (1:2 liquid)
Main Actions	Nervine tonic, tonic, mild laxative
Key Indications	Anxiety, depression
	Impotence, to enhance libido (men and women)
	Nervous dyspepsia, constipation
Major Safety Issues	None known
Key Constituents	Essential oil, resin, arbutin, tannins, tetraphyllin B (a cyanogenic glucoside)
Quality or Adulteration Issues	Other Mexican shrubs which are also called damiana but are unrelated to Turnera, such as Aplopappus venetus, A. discoideus and Chrysactinia mexicana have been substituted

DAN SHEN

Botanical Names(s)	Salvia miltiorrhiza
Part Used	Root
Dose	25 to 50 mL/week (1:2 liquid)
Main Actions	Cardioprotective, hypotensive, anticoagulant, antiplatelet, hepatoprotective, vulnerary, antifibrotic
Key Indications	Angina pectoris, to prevent heart attacks, cardiomyopathy
	Impaired peripheral circulation, Buerger's disease, cerebrovascular disease
	Hypertension, palpitations
	To promote healing of fracture and other wounds
	Hepatitis A, B and C
	Chronic active hepatitis
Other Indications	Acne, scleroderma
	Diabetic neuropathy
	Cancer during chemotherapy (for lymphoma)
	Pancreatitis
Major Safety Issues	Contraindicated in pregnancy and in conjunction with anticoagulant or antiplatelet drugs
Key Constituents	Diterpene diketones (tanshinones)
Quality or Adulteration Issues	No issues identified

DANDELION LEAF

Botanical Names(s)	Taraxacum officinale
Part Used	Leaf
Dose	40 to 80 mL/week (1:1 liquid)
Main Actions	Choleretic, diuretic, mild laxative
Key Indications	Oedema, hypertension
	Digestive liver insufficiency, dyspepsia, constipation
	Gall stones, cholecystitis
Other Indications	Gout

Major Safety Issues	No major issues identified
Key Constituents	Sesquiterpene lactones, triterpenes, coumarins, potassium (about 4%)
Quality or Adulteration Issues	Rarely adulterated with the leaf of Leontodon autumnalis

DANDELION ROOT

Botanical Names(s)	Taraxacum officinale
Part Used	Root
Dose	20 to 40 mL/week (1:2 liquid) 1.5 to 2.0 g/day (tablet)
Main Actions	Bitter tonic, choleretic, mild laxative, antirheumatic, cholagogue, mild diuretic
Key Indications	Digestive liver insufficiency, dyspepsia Flatulent colic, anorexia, constipation Gall stones, cholecystitis, gall bladder dysfunction
Other Indications	Rheumatism Chronic skin disorders
Major Safety Issues	No major issues identified
Key Constituents	Sesquiterpene lactones, taraxacoside, triterpenes, phenolic acids, inulin, potassium (about 2%)
Quality or Adulteration Issues	Rarely adulterated with the root of Cichorium intybus

DEVIL'S CLAW

Botanical Names(s)	Harpagophytum procumbens
Part Used	Root (secondary tuber)
Dose	40 to 80 mL/week (1:2 liquid)
Main Actions	Anti-inflammatory, antirheumatic, analgesic, bitter tonic

Key Indications	Osteoarthritis, rheumatoid arthritis Myalgia, lower back pain Anorexia, dyspepsia (dose: 20 mL/week of 1:2)
Other Indications	Rheumatism, gout
Major Safety Issues	Caution in peptic ulcer
Key Constituents	Iridoid glycosides, primarily harpagoside
Quality or Adulteration Issues	Several adulterants noted but the most common is H. zeyheri

DILL

Botanical Names(s)	Anethum graveolens
Part Used	Fruit
Dose	20 to 40 mL/week (1:2 liquid) 1.2 to 2.3 g/day (tablet)
Main Actions	Carminative, aromatic digestive
Key Indications	Infantile colic, flatulent colic, flatulence, intestinal colic To counter the griping effect of laxative herbs
Major Safety Issues	Caution in gastro-oesophageal reflux
Key Constituents	Essential oil high in carvone
Quality or Adulteration Issues	No issues identified

DONG QUAI

Botanical Names(s)	Angelica sinensis; Angelica polymorpha var sinensis
Part Used	Root
Dose	30 to 60 mL/week (1:2 liquid) 2 to 4 g/day (tablet)
Main Actions	Anti-inflammatory, antianaemic, antiplatelet, uterine tonic, mild laxative, antiarrhythmic

Key Indications	Spasmodic dysmenorrhoea, endometriosis
	Secondary amenorrhoea, menstrual irregularity
	Debility (especially secondary to breastfeeding)
	Impaired peripheral circulation, Buerger's disease, cerebrovascular disease, angina pectoris
	Liver damage
Other Indications	Cardiac arrhythmias, palpitations
Major Safety Issues	Contraindicated in pregnancy (first trimester)
	Caution with warfarin, acute infections and heavy menstruation
Key Constituents	Essential oil (mainly ligustilide and n-butylidene phthalide), ferulic acid, coumarins, phytosterols
Quality or Adulteration Issues	Several adulterants are known including Levisticum officinale

ECHINACEA ROOT

Botanical Names(s)	Echinacea angustifolia and Echinacea purpurea
Part Used	Root
Dose	25 to 60 mL/week (1:2 liquid)
	2.5 to 5.0g/day (tablet)
Main Actions	Immune enhancing, immune modulating, depurative, lymphatic, anti-inflammatory, vulnerary, sialogogue
Key Indications	Acute infections: viral, bacterial or parasitic (all acute doses)
	Chronic infections, swollen lymph glands, splenic enlargement
	Infection prevention, to slow immunological ageing
	Upper and lower respiratory conditions including common cold, influenza, conjunctivitis, sinusitis, nasopharyngeal catarrh, infectious otitis media, pneumonia, pleurisy, bronchiectasis, acute bronchitis, bronchial asthma, pertussis
	Skin conditions including furunculosis, abscesses, ulcers, dermatitis, psoriasis, cellulitis, herpes, shingles
	Gastrointestinal conditions including infection, candidiasis, peptic ulcer, dysentery, cholecystitis, infectious hepatitis
	Urinary tract inflections including cystitis, urethritis, kidney infection
	Dental caries (to prevent), laryngitis, pharyngitis, tonsillitis, mouth ulcers (all liquid preferred)
	Other systemic infections including glandular fever, Ross River virus, mastitis, measles, mumps
Other Indications	Autoimmune disease (controversial)
	Adjunct therapy in cancer including during chemotherapy and radiotherapy, chronic lymphocytic leukaemia, lymphoma
	To promote healing, venomous bites
	Chronic fatigue syndrome, fibromyalgia, post-viral syndromes
Major Safety Issues	Avoid in known allergy. Use cautiously with immunosuppressive drugs
Key Constituents	Alkylamides (isobutylamides), phenolic acid derivatives (cichoric acid)
Quality or Adulteration Issues	Important to use a preparation with a defined content of alkylamides

ELDER BERRY

Botanical Names(s)	Sambucus nigra
Part Used	Berry
Dose	4 to 8 g/day fresh juice (tablet)
Main Actions	Antiviral, immune enhancing, antioxidant
Key Indications	Influenza, common cold and other acute viral infections
	Suitable for children
Major Safety Issues	None known
Key Constituents	Anthocyanins (sambucin, sambucyanin), flavonoids, essential oil, ascorbic acid
Quality or Adulteration Issues	The anthocyanins are unstable in liquid preparations

ELDER FLOWER

Botanical Names(s)	Sambucus nigra
Part Used	Flower
Dose	15 to 40 mL/week (1:2 liquid)
Main Actions	Diaphoretic, anticatarrhal
Key Indications	Common cold, influenza, acute sinusitis (all acute doses)
	Acute infections (with fever), pleurisy, acute bronchitis, measles (all acute doses)
	Chronic sinusitis, hay fever, otitis media (bacterial or serous), pharyngitis, laryngitis, nasopharyngeal catarrh, catarrhal deafness, sinus headache
Other Indications	Asthma (with sinusitis)
Major Safety Issues	None known
Key Constituents	Flavonoids, phenolic acids, triterpenes, essential oil
Quality or Adulteration Issues	Occasional substitution with Sambucus ebulus

ELECAMPANE

Botanical Names(s)	Inula helenium
Part Used	Root
Dose	20 to 40 mL/week (1:2 liquid)
Main Actions	Expectorant, bronchospasmolytic, diaphoretic, antibacterial, spasmolytic
Key Indications	Acute bronchitis, common cold, influenza, pertussis, pneumonia (all acute doses)
	Lower respiratory catarrh, chronic bronchitis, emphysema, bronchiectasis, asthma, bronchial asthma, cough
Major Safety Issues	Avoid in known allergy
Key Constituents	Sesquiterpene lactones of the eudesmanolide type (such as alantolactone, isoalantolactone and their derivatives), essential oil
Quality or Adulteration Issues	Adulteration is very rare, but Belladonna roots are sometimes encountered

EUPHORBIA

Botanical Names(s)	Euphorbia hirta, Euphorbia pilulifera
Part Used	Aerial parts
Dose	5 to 12 mL/week (1:2 liquid)
Main Actions	Expectorant, antiasthmatic, spasmolytic, antiprotozoal
Key Indications	Lower respiratory catarrh, chronic bronchitis, emphysema, bronchial asthma, asthma, laryngitis, pertussis
	Dysentery (amoebic), intestinal parasites (all acute doses)
Other Indications	Intestinal worms (acute doses)
Major Safety Issues	No major issues identified
Key Constituents	Not well defined. Triterpenes, flavonoids, phenolic acid, shikimic acid, choline, tannins

Quality or Adulteration Issues	Can be adulterated with other species of Euphorbia

EVENING PRIMROSE OIL

Botanical Names(s)	Oenothera biennis
Part Used	Fixed oil from the seed
Dose	3 to 6 g fixed oil/day
Main Actions	Anti-inflammatory, antiallergic, hypotensive, nutrient
Key Indications	Inflammatory disorders including dermatitis, rheumatoid arthritis, Raynaud's syndrome, ulcerative colitis Premenstrual syndrome, mastalgia Diabetic neuropathy
Other Indications	Chronic fatigue syndrome, post-viral syndromes Osteoporosis, osteopenia
Major Safety Issues	No major issues identified. Suggested issues with epilepsy have not been proven
Key Constituents	Gamma linolenic acid (8 to 14%), linoleic acid
Quality or Adulteration Issues	No issues identified

EYEBRIGHT

Botanical Names(s)	Euphrasia species
Part Used	Aerial parts
Dose	15 to 30 mL/week (1:2 liquid) 2.0 to 2.6 g/day (tablet)
Main Actions	Anticatarrhal, anti-inflammatory, astringent, mucous membrane tonic
Key Indications	Nasopharyngeal catarrh, chronic sinusitis, hay fever, serous otitis media, pharyngitis, conjunctivitis, blepharitis, catarrhal deafness, sinus headache

	Common cold, acute sinusitis, measles (all acute doses)
Other Indications	Asthma (with sinusitis) Dry eyes
Major Safety Issues	Do not apply herbal tinctures or extracts directly to the eye
Key Constituents	Iridoid glycosides (aucubin, catalpol etc) lignans, flavonoids (quercetin etc)
Quality or Adulteration Issues	Botany is controversial. Medicinal eyebright includes various Euphrasia species (especially E. rostkoviana and E. stricta). Substitution with potentially less active Euphrasia species is possible

FALSE UNICORN

Botanical Names(s)	Chamaelirium luteum, Helonias luteum
Part Used	Root
Dose	15 to 40 mL/week (1:2 liquid)
Main Actions	Uterine tonic, ovarian tonic, oestrogen modulating
Key Indications	Menopausal symptoms Infertility (female), secondary amenorrhoea, erratic ovulation Leucorrhoea, uterine prolapse, cystic hyperplasia of the endometrium, adenomyosis Spasmodic dysmenorrhoea, ovarian pain, ovarian cyst, chronic pelvic inflammation Threatened miscarriage, morning sickness
Other Indications	Menorrhagia, dysfunctional uterine bleeding
Major Safety Issues	Saponins may cause or aggravate gastro-oesophageal reflux
Key Constituents	Not well defined. Saponins (including chamaelirin)

Quality or Adulteration Issues	No issues identified

FENNEL

Botanical Names(s)	Foeniculum vulgare
Part Used	Fruit
Dose	20 to 40 mL/week (1:2 liquid)
	20 to 50 mg essential oil/day
Main Actions	Carminative, spasmolytic, expectorant, orexigenic, galactagogue, antimicrobial, oestrogen modulating
Key Indications	Intestinal colic, flatulence, flatulent colic, infantile colic, dyspepsia
	Anorexia, nausea, diarrhoea
	Difficult lactation, spasmodic dysmenorrhoea, secondary amenorrhoea
	Nasopharyngeal catarrh, acute or chronic bronchitis, bronchial asthma, cough
	Topically for idiopathic hirsutism, conjunctivitis, blepharitis, pharyngitis
Other Indications	Irritable bowel syndrome
	Possibly to assist weight loss
Major Safety Issues	Caution in gastro-oesophageal reflux
Key Constituents	Essential oil (2 to 4%) containing mainly trans-anethole and fenchone, fixed oil, phenolic acids, flavonoids, coumarins, furanocoumarins
Quality or Adulteration Issues	No major issues known

FENUGREEK

Botanical Names(s)	Trigonella foenum-graecum
Part Used	Seed
Dose	15 to 30 mL/week (1:2 liquid)
Main Actions	Hypoglycaemic, hypocholesterolaemic, hypolipidaemic, demulcent, anti-inflammatory, galactagogue, orexigenic
Key Indications	Diabetes
	Dyspepsia, gastritis, gastrointestinal inflammation, anorexia
	Debility, convalescence
	Difficult lactation
Other Indications	Powdered seed for hypercholesterolaemia or elevated triglycerides
Major Safety Issues	Saponins may cause or aggravate gastro-oesophageal reflux. High doses can cause a characteristic body odour
Key Constituents	Steroidal saponins, mucilage, flavonoids, sterols, essential oil, 4-hydroxyisoleucine, trigonelline
Quality or Adulteration Issues	No adulterants known

FEVERFEW

Botanical Names(s)	Tanacetum parthenium
Part Used	Leaf
Dose	7 to 20 mL/week (1:5 liquid)
	150 to 600 mg/day (tablet)
Main Actions	Anti-inflammatory, antiallergic, emmenagogue (high doses), anthelmintic
Key Indications	Prevention and treatment (high doses) of migraine or tension headaches
	Rheumatoid arthritis

Other Indications	Autoimmune disease
	Asthma, dermatitis, hay fever, urticaria
Major Safety Issues	Lower doses during pregnancy. Avoid in known allergy
Key Constituents	Sesquiterpene lactones (eg parthenolide), essential oil
Quality or Adulteration Issues	Some garden varieties may lack adequate levels of parthenolide

FRINGE TREE

Botanical Names(s)	Chionanthus virginicus
Part Used	Root or stem bark
Dose	20 to 40 mL/week (1:2 liquid)
	500 to 800 mg/day (tablet)
Main Actions	Cholagogue, choleretic, mild laxative, antiemetic, depurative
Key Indications	Digestive liver insufficiency, constipation, nausea, dyspepsia
	Gall stones, cholecystitis, gall bladder dysfunction
	Chronic skin disorders
Other Indications	Splenic enlargement, pancreatitis, gastritis, hepatitis, peptic ulcer
	Debility, convalescence
Major Safety Issues	None known
Key Constituents	Pinoresinol and phillyrin and their glucosides, oleuropein, ligustroside
Quality or Adulteration Issues	Use of the stem bark does not compromise activity and is more environmentally sustainable

GARLIC

Botanical Names(s)	Allium sativum
Part Used	Bulb
Dose	40 to 80 mL/week (1:1 fresh plant liquid)
	Allicin-releasing enteric-coated tablets containing 6 to 18 mg of alliin per day
Main Actions	Hypocholesterolaemic, hypotensive, antioxidant, antiplatelet, anthelmintic, antifungal, antiparasitic, antibacterial
Key Indications	Hypercholesterolaemia, elevated triglycerides, hypertension, atherosclerosis
	Common cold, influenza, bronchial asthma, chronic bronchitis, chronic sinusitis, hay fever
	To reduce heavy metal burden
	Gastrointestinal candidiasis, to modify bowel flora
	Intestinal worms
	Peptic ulcer (for Helicobacter)
	Prevention of cardiovascular disease, to prevent heart attacks
	NOTE: For the use of the fresh plant tincture only the first two groupings are relevant, and even for those applications the allicin-releasing tablets are more effective
Major Safety Issues	Contraindicated in known allergy. Use cautiously in conjunction with anticoagulant and antiplatelet drugs and saquinavir. Discontinue 10 days before surgery
Key Constituents	Sulphur compounds (mainly alliin which forms allicin on crushing of the fresh clove), gamma-glutamyl peptides, thioglycosides (scordinins), trace elements (notably selenium)
Quality or Adulteration Issues	Allicin-releasing solid doses should be enteric-coated and tested for enzyme (alliinase) activity

GENTIAN

Botanical Names(s)	Gentiana lutea
Part Used	Root and rhizome
Dose	5 to 15 mL/week (1:2 liquid) 300 to 400 mg/day (tablet)
Main Actions	Bitter tonic, sialagogue, cholagogue
Key Indications	Digestive weakness, hypochlorhydria, anorexia, constipation Flatulence, flatulent colic, intestinal colic, abdominal bloating, nausea Cachexia, debility, convalescence Food allergies/sensitivities
Other Indications	Intestinal worms or parasites (to reduce reinfestation)
Major Safety Issues	Caution in peptic ulcer disease and digestive hyperacidity
Key Constituents	Bitter secoiridoids (amarogentin, gentiopicroside), xanthones, phenolic acids, gentianose (bitter trisaccharide)
Quality or Adulteration Issues	Veratrum album is a toxic adulterant

GINGER

Botanical Names(s)	Zingiber officinale
Part Used	Rhizome
Dose	5 to 15 mL/week (1:2 liquid) 0.9 to 1.2 g/day (tablet)
Main Actions	Antiemetic, carminative, peripheral circulatory stimulant, anti-inflammatory, antiplatelet, diaphoretic, pungent, aromatic digestive
Key Indications	Nausea, morning sickness, travel sickness Digestive weakness, dyspepsia, intestinal colic, abdominal bloating, flatulent colic Acute infections, fever, common cold Acute bronchitis, bronchiectasis, chronic bronchitis, asthma, bronchial asthma Osteoarthritis, rheumatoid arthritis, rheumatism Spasmodic dysmenorrhoea, endometriosis Impaired peripheral circulation, Raynaud's syndrome
Other Indications	Irritable bowel syndrome Food allergies/sensitivities
Major Safety Issues	Caution in peptic ulceration, gallstones, pregnancy and with warfarin
Key Constituents	Pungent principles (gingerols, shogaols), essential oil
Quality or Adulteration Issues	Adulterants include turmeric, cayenne and ferric oxide, especially for powdered ginger

GINKGO

Botanical Names(s)	Ginkgo biloba
Part Used	Leaf
Dose	20 to 40 mL/week (2:1 liquid) 4 to 12 g/day (tablet)
Main Actions	Antioxidant, antiplatelet activating factor (anti-PAF) activity, tissue perfusion enhancing, circulatory stimulant, cognition enhancing, neuroprotective
Key Indications	Alzheimer's disease, vascular dementia (prevention and treatment) Impaired peripheral circulation, gangrene, Raynaud's syndrome Dizziness (of vascular origin) Macular degeneration, impaired retinal blood flow Asthma (anti-PAF) To promote healing

	To improve concentration, memory (short-term memory) or cognitive performance
Other Indications	Tinnitus (controversial)
	Idiopathic hearing loss
	Stroke of recent onset (for recovery)
	Congestive dysmenorrhoea
	Altitude sickness (controversial)
Major Safety Issues	Caution in patients taking anticoagulant drugs, but any risk has been greatly exaggerated
Key Constituents	Flavone glycosides, ginkgolides, bilobalide
Quality or Adulteration Issues	Extract should be standardised for the key constituents and low in ginkgolic acids

GLOBE ARTICHOKE

Botanical Names(s)	Cynara scolymus
Part Used	Leaf
Dose	20 to 55 mL/week (1:2 liquid)
	2.4 to 3.2 g/day (tablet)
Main Actions	Choleretic, hepatoprotective, hepatic trophorestorative, cholagogue, mild bitter tonic, hypocholesterolaemic, hypolipidaemic, antiemetic, diuretic, depurative, diuretic depurative
Key Indications	Digestive liver insufficiency, dyspepsia, irritable bowel syndrome
	Gall stones, cholecystitis, gall bladder dysfunction
	Hypercholesterolaemia, elevated triglycerides
	Nausea, flatulent colic, constipation, flatulence, anorexia, abdominal bloating
Other Indications	Gout, chronic skin conditions
	Food allergies/sensitivities
	Liver damage

Major Safety Issues	Avoid in known allergy
Key Constituents	Caffeic acid derivatives (especially cynarin), sesquiterpene lactones (0.5% to 6%; including cynaropicrin) and flavonoids (0.1% to 1%)
Quality or Adulteration Issues	Occasionally confused with Jerusalem artichoke (Helianthus tuberosus)

GOAT'S RUE

Botanical Names(s)	Galega officinalis
Part Used	Aerial parts
Dose	30 to 60 mL/week (1:2 liquid)
Main Actions	Hypoglycaemic, antidiabetic, galactagogue
Key Indications	Diabetes, insulin resistance
	Difficult lactation
Other Indications	To assist with weight loss, metabolic syndrome X
Major Safety Issues	Caution with patients on antidiabetic drugs or insulin
Key Constituents	Galegine, flavonoids, saponins, traces of chromium
Quality or Adulteration Issues	No adulterants known

GOLDEN ROD

Botanical Names(s)	Solidago virgaurea
Part Used	Aerial parts
Dose	20 to 40 mL/week (1:2 liquid)
	2.0 to 2.6 g/day (tablet)
Main Actions	Anti-inflammatory, diaphoretic, diuretic, anticatarrhal
Key Indications	Nasopharyngeal catarrh, chronic sinusitis, hay fever, serous otitis media, pharyngitis, catarrhal deafness, influenza

	Kidney or bladder stones (treatment and prevention)
	Cystitis, urethritis, nephritis
Other Indications	Rheumatoid arthritis, osteoarthritis
Major Safety Issues	Avoid in known allergy
Key Constituents	Flavonoids, anthocyanidins, saponins, diterpenes, phenolic acids, tannins, essential oil (trace)
Quality or Adulteration Issues	Often adulterated with other species of Solidago

GOLDEN SEAL

Botanical Names(s)	Hydrastis canadensis
Part Used	Root and rhizome
Dose	15 to 30 mL/week (1:3 liquid)
	1.0 to 2.0 g/day (tablet)
Main Actions	Antihaemorrhagic, anticatarrhal, mucous membrane trophorestorative, antimicrobial, antibacterial, bitter tonic, anti-inflammatory, depurative, vulnerary, choleretic, reputed oxytocic
Key Indications	Nasopharyngeal catarrh, chronic sinusitis, hay fever, serous otitis media, pharyngitis, conjunctivitis, blepharitis, catarrhal deafness, sinus headache
	Acne, dermatitis (including topically)
	Peptic ulcer or gastritis (involving Helicobacter), nausea
	Acute gastrointestinal infection with diarrhoea (nonviral), giardiasis, hypertyraminaemia
	Lower respiratory catarrh, bronchiectasis, chronic bronchitis
	Bowel flora, to modify

Other Indications	Convalescence, myalgia
	Menorrhagia
Major Safety Issues	Best avoided during pregnancy and lactation
Key Constituents	Isoquinoline alkaloids (especially beta-hydrastine, berberine, canadine and other alkaloids)
Quality or Adulteration Issues	Due to the price of golden seal, commercial products have regularly been found to be adulterated with berberine-containing herbs such as Coptis and Berberis species

GOTU KOLA

Botanical Names(s)	Centella asiatica
Part Used	Aerial parts
Dose	20 to 40 mL/week (1:1 liquid)
	5 to 8 g/day (tablet)
Main Actions	Healing promoter, vulnerary, anti-inflammatory, adaptogenic, nervine tonic, antifibrotic
Key Indications	To promote healing, to prevent adhesions
	Varicose veins, venous insufficiency, varicose ulcer, haemorrhoids, thrombophlebitis
	Burns, cellulitis, diabetic neuropathy, diabetic ulcer, peptic ulcer, disc prolapse, fractures
	Scleroderma
	Topically for varicose veins, wounds, ulcers, psoriasis, burns, cellulitis, dermatitis, after surgery
Other Indications	Osteopenia, osteoarthritis
	Leprosy
	Restless legs syndrome, night cramps, leg cramps
	Anxiety, to improve concentration or cognitive performance

Major Safety Issues	Avoid in known allergy
Key Constituents	Triterpene saponins (asiaticoside, madecassoside) and their aglycones (asiatic and madecassic acid)
Quality or Adulteration Issues	Unintentional adulteration may occur due to confusion over common names. In Ayurveda both Centella asiatica and Bacopa monnieri are known by the local name "brahmi"

GRAPE SEED

Botanical Names(s)	Vitis vinifera
Part Used	Seed
Dose	Doses of extract containing 85 to 130 mg oligomeric procyanidins/day
Main Actions	Antioxidant, astringent, collagen stabilising, vasoprotective, venotonic
Key Indications	Venous insufficiency, varicose veins, haemorrhoids, varicose ulcer
	Capillary fragility, spider veins, diabetic retinopathy, hypertensive retinopathy, impaired peripheral circulation
	To strengthen connective tissue, to promote healing
	To modify bowel flora
	Following (but not during) radiation therapy for cancer
Other Indications	Macular degeneration, ADHD
	Pancreatitis, chloasma
	To prevent cardiovascular disease or Alzheimer's disease
	Congestive dysmenorrhoea
Major Safety Issues	Take away from mineral supplements

Key Constituents	Catechin and epicatechin and oligomers based on these (oligomeric procyanidins), including dimers (B1, B2 etc) and trimers (C1, C2)
Quality or Adulteration Issues	No adulterants known

GRAVEL ROOT

Botanical Names(s)	Eupatorium purpureum
Part Used	Rhizome and root
Dose	15 to 30 mL/week (1:2 liquid)
Main Actions	Antilithic, diuretic, diuretic depurative
Key Indications	Kidney stones or bladder stones (treatment and prevention)
	Dysuria, prostatitis, haematuria
Other Indications	Gout, rheumatism
	Urinary incontinence
Major Safety Issues	None known
Key Constituents	Not well defined. Essential oil, resin, flavonoids (euparin)
Quality or Adulteration Issues	Can be adulterated with other species of Eupatorium

GREATER CELANDINE

Botanical Names(s)	Chelidonium majus
Part Used	Aerial parts
Dose	7 to 15 mL/week (1:2 liquid)
Main Actions	Choleretic, cholagogue, spasmolytic, mild laxative, anti-inflammatory, antiviral (topically), vulnerary (topically)
Key Indications	Digestive liver insufficiency, dyspepsia, irritable bowel syndrome
	Gall stones, cholecystitis, gall bladder dysfunction

	Migraine headache, psoriasis
	Topically for warts
Major Safety Issues	Avoid exceeding recommended doses and long-term use due to the risk of idiosyncratic liver damage
Key Constituents	Isoquinoline alkaloids (sanguinarine, chelidonine, berberine, coptisine)
Quality or Adulteration Issues	No adulterants known

GREEN TEA

Botanical Names(s)	Camellia sinensis
Part Used	Leaf
Dose	Doses of extract containing 170 to 250 mg of catechins/day
Main Actions	Antioxidant, astringent, antibacterial, antiviral, hypocholesterolaemic, diuretic, anticarcinogenic
Key Indications	To prevent cancer, Alzheimer's disease or cardiovascular disease
	To modify bowel flora
	To assist with weight loss
	Adjunctive treatment in cancer
	To slow the ageing process
Other Indications	Chronic lymphocytic leukaemia
	Hypercholesterolaemia
	Haemochromatosis
Major Safety Issues	Take away from mineral supplements. Alcoholic extracts have been implicated in liver damage. Excessive doses may aggravate insomnia and palpitations
Key Constituents	Hydrolysable tannins (collectively known as green tea catechins, including epigallocatechin gallate), methylxanthines (mainly caffeine), flavonoids, triterpenoid saponins, theanine, phenolic acids, theaflavins
Quality or Adulteration Issues	Preparations should contain aqueous extracts and not be decaffeinated

GRINDELIA

Botanical Names(s)	Grindelia camporum; Grindelia robusta
Part Used	Aerial parts
Dose	10 to 20 mL/week (1:2 liquid)
	0.9 to 1.2 g/day (tablet)
Main Actions	Expectorant, bronchospasmolytic
Key Indications	Asthma, bronchial asthma, pertussis, chronic bronchitis
	Cough, upper and lower respiratory catarrh
Major Safety Issues	No major issues identified
Key Constituents	Diterpenes (resin), acetylenic compounds, flavonoids, triterpenoid saponins, phenolic acids, essential oil
Quality or Adulteration Issues	No adulterants known

GROUND IVY

Botanical Names(s)	Glechoma hederacea; Nepeta hederacea
Part Used	Aerial parts
Dose	20 to 40 mL/week (1:2 liquid)
Main Actions	Anticatarrhal, mild expectorant, astringent
Key Indications	Nasopharyngeal catarrh, chronic sinusitis, hay fever, serous otitis media, pharyngitis, catarrhal deafness
	Cough, chronic bronchitis

Major Safety Issues	None known
Key Constituents	Not well defined. Flavonoids, triterpenoids, phenolic acids, tannins, essential oil (trace), marrubiin, amino acids
Quality or Adulteration Issues	No issues identified

GYMNEMA

Botanical Names(s)	Gymnema sylvestre
Part Used	Leaf
Dose	25 to 75 mL/week (1:1 liquid)
	4 to 16 g/day (tablet)
Main Actions	Antidiabetic, hypoglycaemic, hypocholesterolaemic, hypolipidaemic, antiobesity
Key Indications	Diabetes, insulin resistance
	Metabolic syndrome X, to assist with weight loss
	Sweet craving, dysglycaemia (lower doses)
	Hypercholesterolaemia, elevated triglycerides
Major Safety Issues	Saponins may cause or aggravate gastro-oesophageal reflux
Key Constituents	Saponins (gymnemic acids, gymnemasaponins)
Quality or Adulteration Issues	No adulterants known

HAWTHORN

Botanical Names(s)	Crataegus monogyna, Crataegus laevigata
Part Used	Leaves with flowers, berries or both
Dose	20 to 50 mL/week (berry, 1:2 liquid)
	20 to 40 mL/week (leaf, 1:2 liquid)
	3 to 4 g/day (tablet)
Main Actions	Cardioprotective, mild cardiotonic, hypotensive, peripheral vasodilator, antiarrhythmic, antioxidant, mild astringent, collagen stabilising
Key Indications	Mild congestive cardiac failure, cardiac arrhythmias
	Angina pectoris, to prevent heart attacks, cardiomyopathy
	Impaired peripheral circulation, Buerger's disease
	Hypertension, palpitations
	Mild anxiety
Other Indications	Menopausal symptoms (hot flushes/flashes)
Major Safety Issues	No major issues identified. Caution with digoxin, although negative interaction has not been established. Take away from mineral supplements, thiamine or alkaloids
Key Constituents	Oligomeric procyanidins (1% to 3%), mainly procyanidin B-2, flavonoids (1% to 2%), including quercetin glycosides (hyperoside, rutin) and flavone-C-glycosides (vitexin). The flowers contain the highest levels of flavonoids and the leaves contain the highest levels of oligomeric procyanidins
Quality or Adulteration Issues	No adulterants known

HEMIDESMUS

Botanical Names(s)	Hemidesmus indicus
Part Used	Root
Dose	25 to 60 mL/week (1:2 liquid)
	1.5 to 2.5 g/day (tablet)
Main Actions	Depurative, diaphoretic, immune depressant
Key Indications	Autoimmune disease

	Rheumatoid arthritis, multiple sclerosis Chronic skin disorders
Major Safety Issues	None known
Key Constituents	Not well defined. Essential oil, triterpenoid saponins. Does not contain coumarin, despite the root's vanilla-like odour
Quality or Adulteration Issues	No adulterants known

HOPS

Botanical Names(s)	Humulus lupulus
Part Used	Strobile
Dose	10 to 20 mL/week (1:2 liquid)
Main Actions	Hypnotic, mild sedative, spasmolytic, anaphrodisiac (male), bitter tonic, oestrogen modulating
Key Indications	Sleep maintenance or sleep onset insomnia Anxiety, excitability, restlessness, panic attacks Anorexia, nervous dyspepsia Neuralgia, tension headache, trigeminal neuralgia Excessive libido in men
Other Indications	Menopausal symptoms Irritable bowel syndrome Androgen excess
Major Safety Issues	Best avoided with oestrogen-sensitive breast cancer. Traditionally contraindicated in depression
Key Constituents	Phloroglucinol derivatives (bitter resin containing humulone, lupulone etc), essential oil, flavonoids, phenolic acids, oestrogenic chalcone (xanthohumol)

Quality or Adulteration Issues	Rarely contaminated with wild hops which is less effective

HORSECHESTNUT

Botanical Names(s)	Aesculus hippocastanum
Part Used	Seed
Dose	15 to 35 mL/week (1:2 liquid) 2.4 to 3.6 g/day (tablet)
Main Actions	Venotonic, antioedema, anti-inflammatory
Key Indications	Venous insufficiency Varicose veins, haemorrhoids Varicose ulcer Lymphoedema Deep vein thrombosis (to reduce risk) Disorders where local tissue oedema may be involved in nerve compression such as trigeminal neuralgia, Bell's palsy, sciatica, disc lesions, carpal tunnel syndrome Topically for haematoma, contusions, sprains
Other Indications	Restless legs syndrome, leg cramps, night cramps Spider veins, capillary fragility, bruises, easy bruising
Major Safety Issues	Saponins can cause or aggravate gastro-oesophageal reflux. Should not be applied directly to broken or ulcerated skin
Key Constituents	Triterpenoid saponins (aescin), flavonoids
Quality or Adulteration Issues	No adulterants known. Best to use as an enteric-coated solid dose preparation to avoid reflux

HORSERADISH

Botanical Names(s)	Armoracia rusticana
Part Used	Root
Dose	25 to 50 mL/week (1:2 liquid)
Main Actions	Pungent, anticatarrhal, counterirritant, circulatory and metabolic stimulant
Key Indications	Nasopharyngeal catarrh, chronic sinusitis, sinus headache, hay fever
	Acute sinusitis, common cold
Other Indications	Topically for osteoarthritis
Major Safety Issues	Topical or internal use may cause discomfort and burning. High doses best avoided in peptic ulcers, pregnancy and hypothyroidism
Key Constituents	Glucosinolates, coumarins, phenolic acids
Quality or Adulteration Issues	No adulterants known

HORSETAIL

Botanical Names(s)	Equisetum arvense
Part Used	Aerial parts
Dose	15 to 40 mL/week (1:2 liquid)
Main Actions	Mild diuretic, astringent, styptic, antihaemorrhagic
Key Indications	Cystitis, urethritis, haematuria, dysuria
	Prostatitis (acute or chronic), benign prostatic hyperplasia (BPH)
	Nocturnal enuresis
Other Indications	Topically for wounds
	Urinary incontinence
Major Safety Issues	No major issues identified
Key Constituents	Flavonoids, caffeic acid esters, alkaloids (traces), silica (of doubtful bioavailability)
Quality or Adulteration Issues	Adulteration can occur with other species of Equisetum which may be mildly toxic

HYDRANGEA

Botanical Names(s)	Hydrangea arborescens
Part Used	Root
Dose	15 to 50 mL/week (1:2 liquid)
Main Actions	Diuretic, antilithic, antiprostatic
Key Indications	Prostatitis (acute or chronic), benign prostatic hyperplasia (BPH)
	Kidney or bladder stones, dysuria, cystitis, urethritis
Major Safety Issues	None known
Key Constituents	Not well defined. Resin, coumarins, saponins
Quality or Adulteration Issues	No adulterants known

HYSSOP

Botanical Names(s)	Hyssopus officinalis
Part Used	Aerial parts
Dose	15 to 30 mL/week (1:2 liquid)
Main Actions	Expectorant, carminative, spasmolytic, diaphoretic, mild sedative
Key Indications	Nasopharyngeal catarrh, asthma, bronchial asthma, chronic bronchitis
	Common cold, fever, acute bronchitis
Other Indications	Epilepsy (petit mal)
	Topically as a gargle for pharyngitis
Major Safety Issues	Best avoided in pregnancy
Key Constituents	Essential oil, flavonoids (diosmin), phenylpropanoids
Quality or Adulteration Issues	No adulterants known

INULA RACEMOSA

Botanical Names(s)	Inula racemosa
Part Used	Root
Dose	30 to 60 mL/week (1:2 liquid)
Main Actions	Spasmolytic, hypotensive, bronchospasmolytic
Key Indications	Angina pectoris
	Asthma, bronchial asthma
	Chronic bronchitis with cardiac complications
	Given the similarities in phytochemistry, elecampane can possibly be substituted should Inula racemosa be unavailable
Major Safety Issues	Avoid in known allergy
Key Constituents	Sesquiterpene lactones of the eudesmanolide type (alantolactone etc), essential oil
Quality or Adulteration Issues	No adulterants known

JAMAICA DOGWOOD

Botanical Names(s)	Piscidia erythrina; Piscidia piscipula
Part Used	Root bark
Dose	20 to 40 mL/week (1:2 liquid)
Main Actions	Analgesic, spasmolytic, mild sedative
Key Indications	Pain management for nerve-generated pain (acute doses as required)
	Neuralgia, sciatica, trigeminal neuralgia, toothache, tension headache (all acute doses as required)
	Insomnia
	Anxiety, emotional stress
	Spasmodic dysmenorrhoea, migraine headache
Major Safety Issues	Contraindicated in pregnancy, bradycardia or cardiac insufficiency

Key Constituents	Isoflavonoids, rotenoids, organic acids, tannins
Quality or Adulteration Issues	No adulterants known

JUNIPER

Botanical Names(s)	Juniperus communis
Part Used	Cone berries
Dose	10 to 20 mL/week (1:2 liquid)
Main Actions	Urinary antiseptic, mild diuretic, carminative, anti-inflammatory
Key Indications	Cystitis, urethritis, dysuria (all acute doses)
	Recurrent cystitis
	Rheumatism, osteoarthritis
Other Indications	Gout
	Acute prostatitis (acute doses)
Major Safety Issues	Contraindicated in pregnancy. The reputed contraindication in renal inflammation probably relates to effects from the unripe berries
Key Constituents	Essential oil, diterpenoids (resin), flavonoids, fatty alcohol
Quality or Adulteration Issues	Adulteration with unripe berries or the needle-like leaves increases the possibility of adverse effects

KAVA

Botanical Names(s)	Piper methysticum
Part Used	Root
Dose	6 to 9 g/day (tablet)
Main Actions	Anxiolytic, hypnotic, anticonvulsant, mild sedative, skeletal muscle relaxant, spasmolytic, local anaesthetic, mild analgesic, antipruritic (topically)

Key Indications	Anxiety, excitability, panic attacks, emotional stress
	Insomnia (sleep onset, sleep maintenance)
	Menopausal symptoms
	Toothache, pharyngitis (both topically)
	Leg cramps, muscular tension
Other Indications	Tension headache, neuralgia, chronic prostatitis, prostatism
Major Safety Issues	Caution in Parkinson's disease, pregnancy and lactation. May rarely cause liver damage
Key Constituents	Kava lactones (or pyrones), mainly kavain (or kawain), dihydrokavain, methysticin
Quality or Adulteration Issues	Because of the association with liver damage the aqueous extract (as a tablet) or powdered herb is preferred

KOLA NUT

Botanical Names(s)	Cola nitida; Cola vera
Part Used	Seed
Dose	10 to 25 mL/week (1:1 liquid)
Main Actions	CNS stimulant, thymoleptic, mild diuretic
Key Indications	Fatigue, debility (short-term use)
Other Indications	Depression (with general muscular weakness)
Major Safety Issues	Contraindicated in hypertension, peptic ulcers, insomnia and caffeine sensitivity
Key Constituents	Caffeine (1.5 to 2.5%), theobromine, tannins
Quality or Adulteration Issues	No adulterants known

KOREAN GINSENG

Botanical Names(s)	Panax ginseng
Part Used	Main and lateral roots
Dose	7 to 40 mL/week (1:2 liquid)
	300 to 500 mg/day (tablet)
Main Actions	Adaptogenic, tonic, immune modulating, cardiotonic, male tonic, cancer preventative, cognition enhancing
Key Indications	Debility, emaciation, cachexia, chronic immune deficiency
	Fatigue, physical stress, convalescence, failure to thrive
	To improve physical and mental performance and concentration
	Cancer during chemotherapy or radiotherapy, to prevent cancer
	Cancer (adjunct treatment)
	Impotence, male infertility
	Type 2 diabetes
	Mild congestive cardiac failure
	Menopausal symptoms
	To slow ageing, as a tonic for the elderly
	Post-viral syndromes, chronic fatigue syndrome, fibromyalgia
Other Indications	HIV/AIDS (as adjunct treatment)
	ADHD
	Drug abuse or addiction
Major Safety Issues	Caution in acute states (such as mania, asthma attacks, infection, nose bleeds, menorrhagia) and with CNS stimulants (caffeine, amphetamines). Overstimulation may occur. Controversial in hypertension. Best avoided with warfarin and MAOI antidepressants such as phenelzine

Key Constituents	Ginsenosides, essential oil, polyacetylenes, peptides, lipids
Quality or Adulteration Issues	The main and lateral roots can be adulterated with the inferior hair roots

LADIES MANTLE

Botanical Names(s)	Alchemilla vulgaris
Part Used	Aerial parts
Dose	25 to 50 mL/week (1:2 liquid) 2.0 to 2.6 g/day (tablet)
Main Actions	Astringent, antihaemorrhagic, anti-inflammatory
Key Indications	Menorrhagia, metrorrhagia Endometriosis, menopausal symptoms
Other Indications	Diarrhoea, gastrointestinal infection Leucorrhoea, pruritis vulvae (both topically)
Major Safety Issues	No major issues identified
Key Constituents	Not well defined. Ellagitannins (agrimoniin), flavonoids, phytosterols
Quality or Adulteration Issues	No adulterants known

LAVENDER

Botanical Names(s)	Lavandula officinalis; Lavandula angustifolia
Part Used	Flower
Dose	15 to 30 mL/week (1:2 liquid)
Main Actions	Carminative, spasmolytic, antidepressant, anxiolytic
Key Indications	Anxiety, insomnia, excitability, nervous dyspepsia Mild depression Flatulent colic, intestinal colic

Other Indications	Irritable bowel syndrome Tension headache
Major Safety Issues	Avoid in known allergy
Key Constituents	Essential oil (mainly linalyl acetate and linalool)
Quality or Adulteration Issues	Adulteration can occur with inferior species of Lavender

LEMON BALM

Botanical Names(s)	Melissa officinalis
Part Used	Aerial parts
Dose	20 to 40 mL/week (1:2 liquid)
Main Actions	Carminative, spasmolytic, mild sedative, diaphoretic, TSH antagonist, antiviral (topically)
Key Indications	Insomnia, anxiety, irritability, depression Infantile colic, flatulence, flatulent colic, intestinal colic, nervous dyspepsia Topically for herpes infections
Other Indications	Fever, common cold, influenza Irritable bowel syndrome
Major Safety Issues	No major issues known
Key Constituents	Essential oil (containing citronellal, citral), phenolic acids, flavonoids
Quality or Adulteration Issues	Adulteration occasionally occurs with Nepeta cataria var citriodora

LICORICE

Botanical Names(s)	Glycyrrhiza glabra
Part Used	Root
Dose	10 to 40 mL/week (1:1 liquid) 2.0 to 3.0 g/day (tablet)

Main Actions	Anti-inflammatory, mucoprotective, adrenal tonic, expectorant, demulcent, mild laxative, anticariogenic, antitussive
Key Indications	Peptic ulcer, gastritis, gastro-oesophageal reflux
	Adrenal depletion, physical stress, Addison's disease
	Polycystic ovary syndrome, infertility (female), androgen excess (female)
	Acute or chronic bronchitis, asthma, cough, bronchial asthma
	Constipation
	Topically for mouth ulcers, dermatitis, melasma, herpes, acne
Other Indications	Acute or recurrent cystitis
	To support withdrawal from corticosteroid drugs
Major Safety Issues	Best not to exceed 30 mL per week for high glycyrrhizin liquid extracts. Contraindicated (except in low doses or for deglycyrrhinized preparations) in hypertension, hypokalaemia, oedema, congestive heart failure. Caution in the elderly or those with cardiac, renal or hepatic disease and with digoxin, diuretics or laxatives
Key Constituents	Glycyrrhizin, glycyrrhetinic acid, flavonoids (liquiritin, isoliquiritin)
Quality or Adulteration Issues	Other species of Glycyrrhiza

LIME FLOWERS

Botanical Names(s)	Tilia cordata; Tilia platyphyllos; Tilia x europea
Part Used	Flower
Dose	15 to 30 mL/week (1:2 liquid)
Main Actions	Diaphoretic, spasmolytic, peripheral vasodilator, mild sedative
Key Indications	Fever, common cold, influenza
	Angina, palpitations, hypertension
	Anxiety, insomnia, tension headache
Other Indications	Migraine headache
Major Safety Issues	Avoid in known allergy. May reduce iron absorption when taken concurrently
Key Constituents	Not well defined. Flavonoids, phenolic acids, mucilage, tannins, essential oil (trace)
Quality or Adulteration Issues	Many other species of Tilia can be found as adulterants

LOMATIUM

Botanical Names(s)	Lomatium dissectum
Part Used	Root
Dose	15 to 40 mL/week (1:2 liquid)
Main Actions	Antiviral (reputedly)
Key Indications	Common cold, influenza, herpes simplex infection
	Post-viral syndromes, chronic fatigue syndrome
Major Safety Issues	Continued use may cause a skin rash, presumably allergic
Key Constituents	Essential oil, flavonoids, coumarin, glycosides, tetronic acids
Quality or Adulteration Issues	No issues identified

MARSHMALLOW ROOT

Botanical Names(s)	Althaea officinalis
Part Used	Root
Dose	20 to 40 mL/week (1:5 liquid)

Main Actions	Demulcent, reflex demulcent, emollient
Key Indications	Gastro-oesophageal reflux, peptic ulcer, gastritis
	Asthma, acute or chronic bronchitis, cough
	Cystitis, urethritis, dysuria
	Inflammation of the gastrointestinal tract, irritable bowel syndrome, constipation, ulcerative colitis
	Topically for abscesses, furunculosis, leg ulcer, pharyngitis, laryngitis, varicose ulcer, burns
Other Indications	To modify bowel flora
Major Safety Issues	Best taken away from prescribed drugs as it may retard their absorption
Key Constituents	Mucilage, flavonoids, phenolic acids, starch
Quality or Adulteration Issues	Use of the glycetract is preferred to the tincture as it better extracts the mucilage

MEADOWSWEET

Botanical Names(s)	Filipendula ulmaria
Part Used	Aerial parts
Dose	20 to 40 mL/week (1:2 liquid)
	1.5 to 3 g/day (tablet)
Main Actions	Antacid, anti-inflammatory, mild urinary antiseptic, astringent, mucoprotective
Key Indications	Peptic ulcer, gastritis, gastro-oesophageal reflux
	Dyspepsia, diarrhoea, irritable bowel syndrome, gastrointestinal inflammation
Other Indications	Cystitis, urethritis, dysuria
	Rheumatism, myalgia
	Fever, common cold

Major Safety Issues	Use cautiously with warfarin. Avoid in known salicylate sensitivity. Take away from mineral supplements, thiamine or alkaloids
Key Constituents	Various phenolic glycosides which are salicylate derivates (eg spiraein), essential oil (mainly salicylaldehyde), flavonoids, tannins
Quality or Adulteration Issues	Adulteration with other species of Filipendula

MEXICAN VALERIAN

Botanical Names(s)	Valeriana edulis
Part Used	Root and rhizome
Dose	20 to 40 mL/week (1:2 liquid)
	2.0 to 4.0 g/day (tablet)
Main Actions	Anxiolytic, mild sedative, hypnotic, spasmolytic
Key Indications	Anxiety, excitability, irritability
	Insomnia, panic attacks, emotional stress
Other Indications	Hypertension, tension headache
Major Safety Issues	No major issues identified
Key Constituents	Iridoid compounds known as valepotriates (valtrate, isovaltrate etc), essential oil
Quality or Adulteration Issues	Other species of Valerian can be adulterants

MISTLETOE

Botanical Names(s)	Viscum album
Part Used	Aerial parts
Dose	20 to 40 mL/week (1:2 liquid)
Main Actions	Hypotensive, peripheral vasodilator, mild sedative
Key Indications	Hypertension, angina pectoris
	Epilepsy, excitability

Other Indications	Tachycardia
Major Safety Issues	No major issues identified
Key Constituents	Not well defined. Phenylpropanoids, lignans, polypeptides, amino acids
Quality or Adulteration Issues	The anticancer activity of mistletoe only applies for fresh plant preparations administered by injection

MOTHERWORT

Botanical Names(s)	Leonurus cardiaca
Part Used	Aerial parts
Dose	15 to 25 mL/week (1:2 liquid)
Main Actions	Nervine tonic, cardiotonic, hypotensive, antiarrhythmic, antithyroid, spasmolytic, emmenagogue
Key Indications	Hyperthyroidism (for the cardiac symptoms) Palpitations, nervous tachycardia Secondary amenorrhoea, dysmenorrhoea, ovarian pain
Other Indications	Anxiety, neuralgia
Major Safety Issues	Use with caution during pregnancy, but adverse effects are unlikely on current information
Key Constituents	Alkaloids (L-stachydrine, leonurine), iridoids, diterpenoids, flavonoids, caffeic acid derivatives, tannins
Quality or Adulteration Issues	Other species of Leonurus are potential adulterants as the correct species is often confused by herb growers

MUGWORT

Botanical Names(s)	Artemisia vulgaris
Part Used	Aerial parts
Dose	15 to 30 mL/week (1:2 liquid)
Main Actions	Emmenagogue, choleretic, orexigenic, anthelmintic
Key Indications	Digestive weakness, anorexia, nervous dyspepsia
Other Indications	Secondary amenorrhoea, dysmenorrhoea Intestinal worms
Major Safety Issues	Best avoided in pregnancy and lactation
Key Constituents	Phenolic acids, coumarins, flavonoids, essential oil, sesquiterpene lactones
Quality or Adulteration Issues	No adulterants known

MULLEIN

Botanical Names(s)	Verbascum thapsus
Part Used	Leaf
Dose	30 to 60 mL/week (1:2 liquid) 1.5 to 2.0 g/day (tablet)
Main Actions	Expectorant, demulcent, anticatarrhal, vulnerary
Key Indications	Acute bronchitis, chronic bronchitis, bronchiectasis, tracheitis, lower respiratory catarrh, cough Common cold, influenza, pharyngitis
Other Indications	Peptic ulcer, diarrhoea Topically for wounds, haemorrhoids, earache (infused oil)
Major Safety Issues	None known

Key Constituents	Iridoid glycosides, flavonoids, saponins, triterpenes
Quality or Adulteration Issues	No adulterants known

MYRRH

Botanical Names(s)	Commiphora molmol; Commiphora myrrha
Part Used	Oleogum resin
Dose	10 to 30 mL/week (1:5 liquid)
Main Actions	Astringent, antimicrobial, antibacterial, anti-inflammatory, vulnerary, anthelmintic, lymphatic
Key Indications	Intestinal worms or parasites (high doses for short periods) Chronic bronchitis, common cold, nasopharyngeal catarrh Topically for mouth ulcers, pharyngitis, tonsillitis, wounds, gingivitis, halitosis
Major Safety Issues	Long-term intake and use in pregnancy are best avoided. Can cause contact dermatitis and allergic reaction after oral ingestion
Key Constituents	Essential oil (mainly sesquiterpenes), resin (including commiphoric acids), gum
Quality or Adulteration Issues	Gum arabic and other species of Commiphora are known adulterants

NETTLE LEAF

Botanical Names(s)	Urtica dioica; Urtica urens
Part Used	Leaf
Dose	15 to 40 mL/week (1:2 liquid)
Main Actions	Antirheumatic, antiallergic, depurative, styptic (haemostatic)
Key Indications	Hay fever, dermatitis, urticaria
	Osteoarthritis, rheumatism, rheumatoid arthritis
Other Indications	Uterine or gastrointestinal bleeding, epistaxis Acne
Major Safety Issues	Rare allergic reactions may occur
Key Constituents	Not well defined. Flavonoids, amines, silicic acid, rich in chlorophyll
Quality or Adulteration Issues	Rare adulteration with Belladonna has occurred

NETTLE ROOT

Botanical Names(s)	Urtica dioica; Urtica urens
Part Used	Root
Dose	30 to 60 mL/week (1:2 liquid) 2.0 to 2.7 g/day (capsule)
Main Actions	Antiprostatic
Key Indications	Benign prostatic hyperplasia (BPH) Chronic prostatitis
Major Safety Issues	None known
Key Constituents	Lignans, sterols, hydroxyfatty acids, lectins, fatty alcohols
Quality or Adulteration Issues	No adulterants known

OATS, GREEN

Botanical Names(s)	Avena sativa
Part Used	Aerial parts
Dose	20 to 40 mL/week (1:2 liquid)
Main Actions	Nervine tonic, anxiolytic
Key Indications	Fatigue (especially nervous) Drug abuse/addiction (controversial) Anxiety, insomnia, mild depression

Major Safety Issues	None known
Key Constituents	Not well defined
Quality or Adulteration Issues	No adulterants known

OATS, SEED

Botanical Names(s)	Avena sativa
Part Used	Seed
Dose	20 to 40 mL/week (1:1 liquid)
Main Actions	Nervine tonic, tonic, thymoleptic
Key Indications	Debility, convalescence Fatigue (especially nervous), mild depression Drug abuse/addiction (controversial) Insomnia (sleep maintenance) Topically (as a decoction) for dermatitis
Other Indications	Menopausal symptoms
Major Safety Issues	None known
Key Constituents	Not well defined. Triterpenoid saponins (avenacosides), alkaloids(eg gramine, trigonelline), flavonoids, starch, beta-glucan
Quality or Adulteration Issues	No adulterants known

OLIVE LEAF

Botanical Names(s)	Olea europaea
Part Used	Leaf
Dose	25 to 50 mL/week (1:2 liquid)
Main Actions	Hypotensive, antioxidant, bitter tonic
Key Indications	Hypertension, angina pectoris
Other Indications	Note that the reputed uses of olive leaf as an immunostimulant or systemic antimicrobial or antiviral has no traditional support nor evidence from well-designed clinical trials
Major Safety Issues	None known
Key Constituents	Iridoid glycosides (mainly oleuropein), flavonoids
Quality or Adulteration Issues	No adulterants known

OREGANO

Botanical Names(s)	Origanum vulgare
Part Used	Aerial parts
Dose	230 to 450 mg/day (essential oil)
Main Actions	Antifungal, antibacterial, antioxidant
Key Indications	Gastrointestinal candidiasis To modify bowel flora Peptic ulcer for Helicobacter Chronic bronchitis, bronchiectasis, bronchial asthma
Major Safety Issues	Avoid in known allergy
Key Constituents	Essential oil containing mainly phenols (carvacrol, thymol), phenolic acids
Quality or Adulteration Issues	Best to use an enteric-coated preparation to maximise the impact on bowel flora

OREGON GRAPE

Botanical Names(s)	Mahonia aquifolium; Berberis aquifolium
Part Used	Root and rhizome
Dose	25 to 50 mL/week (1:2 liquid) 1.4 to 1.8 g/day (tablet)
Main Actions	Depurative, anti-inflammatory, antimicrobial

Key Indications	Chronic skin disorders, psoriasis, acne, dermatitis
	Topically for psoriasis, acne
Major Safety Issues	Best avoided in pregnancy and lactation
Key Constituents	Alkaloids including magnoflorine, berberine, jatrorrhizine
Quality or Adulteration Issues	No adulterants known

PAEONIA (WHITE PEONY)

Botanical Names(s)	Paeonia lactiflora
Part Used	Root
Dose	30 to 60 mL/week (1:2 liquid)
	2.2 to 4.2 g/day (tablet)
Main Actions	Spasmolytic, mild skeletal muscle relaxant, anticonvulsant, anti-inflammatory, cognition enhancer, antiallergic, oestrogen modulating
Key Indications	Polycystic ovary syndrome, endometriosis, fibroids, adenomyosis, androgen excess, oestrogen excess
	Epilepsy, to improve memory, concentration or mental performance
	Spasmodic dysmenorrhoea, menstrual irregularity, leucorrhoea, menorrhagia
Other Indications	Leg cramps, angina pectoris, migraine headache
	Alzheimer's disease
Major Safety Issues	No major issues identified
Key Constituents	Paeoniflorin, benzoylpaeoniflorin, albiflorin, paeonilactones
Quality or Adulteration Issues	The bleached root contains sulphite derivatives of paeoniflorin and should be avoided

PASQUE FLOWER

Botanical Names(s)	Anemone pulsatilla; Pulsatilla vulgaris
Part Used	Aerial parts
Dose	3 to 10 mL/week (1:2 liquid)
Main Actions	Spasmolytic, analgesic
Key Indications	Painful or inflamed conditions of the male or female reproductive tract such as spasmodic dysmenorrhoea, ovarian pain, orchitis
Other Indications	Insomnia, excitability, tension headache
Major Safety Issues	Use cautiously in children. Contraindicated in known allergy, pregnancy and lactation
Key Constituents	Not well defined. Anemonin, triterpenoid saponins, tannins, essential oil
Quality or Adulteration Issues	The danger of adulteration arises from other more toxic species such as Pulsatilla patens

PASSIONFLOWER

Botanical Names(s)	Passiflora incarnata
Part Used	Aerial parts
Dose	20 to 40 mL/week (1:2 liquid)
	1.5 to 2.5 g/day (tablet)
Main Actions	Anxiolytic, spasmolytic, mild sedative, hypnotic
Key Indications	Sleep onset or maintenance insomnia
	Anxiety, excitability, irritability
	Nervous tachycardia, tension headache, palpitations
Other Indications	Drug abuse/addiction
	Trigeminal neuralgia, spasmodic dysmenorrhoea, asthma, epilepsy
Major Safety Issues	No major issues identified

Key Constituents	Flavonoids, especially flavone-C-glycosides such as isovitexin and derivatives, maltol, isomaltol, traces of harmane alkaloids
Quality or Adulteration Issues	Important to avoid the white-flowered variety which has a differing phytochemical makeup. Can also be adulterated with other Passiflora species

PAU D'ARCO

Botanical Names(s)	Tabebuia avellanedae; Tabebuia impetiginosa
Part Used	Bark
Dose	25 to 50 mL/week (1:2 liquid) 1.5 to 2.5 g/day (tablet)
Main Actions	Immune enhancing, antitumour, antibacterial, antifungal, antiparasitic, depurative
Key Indications	Adjunct therapy in cancer Intestinal parasites or candida Topically for fungal infections
Major Safety Issues	Avoid using in pregnancy and with anticoagulant drugs such as warfarin
Key Constituents	Naphthoquinones such as beta-lapachone and lapachol, iridoids, anthraquinones
Quality or Adulteration Issues	Other species of Tabebuia are adulterants, which may cause adverse effects

PELARGONIUM

Botanical Names(s)	Pelargonium sidoides; Pelargonium reniforme
Part Used	Root
Dose	20 to 40 mL/week (1:5 liquid)
Main Actions	Antibacterial, immune modulating, expectorant, antifungal
Key Indications	Acute bronchitis, acute tonsillitis, acute pharyngitis, infectious otitis media

	Acute sinusitis, common cold Especially proven in clinical trials involving children
Other Indications	Tuberculosis, bronchiectasis, pneumonia, pleurisy, chronic bronchitis, bronchial asthma
Major Safety Issues	Take away from mineral supplements
Key Constituents	Highly oxygenated coumarins, flavan-3-ols, procyanidins, gallic acid derivatives, essential oil
Quality or Adulteration Issues	Other species of Pelargonium are potential adulterants. The tincture used should closely match the phytochemical profile of that used in the European clinical trials

PEPPERMINT

Botanical Names(s)	Mentha x piperita
Part Used	Leaf
Dose	10 to 30 mL/week (1:2 liquid)
Main Actions	Spasmolytic, carminative, cholagogue, antiemetic, antitussive, antimicrobial (internally and topically), mild sedative, diaphoretic, analgesic (topically), antipruritic (topically)
Key Indications	Dyspepsia, intestinal colic, flatulence, flatulent colic, infantile colic Irritable bowel syndrome (especially the essential oil) Gall bladder dysfunction, gall stones Gastritis, nausea, morning sickness Common cold, influenza, cough, nasopharyngeal catarrh, sinus headache
Other Indications	Topically for tension headache, pruritis, osteoarthritis, neuralgia (especially the essential oil) To inhibit lactation

Major Safety Issues	Contraindicated in gastro-oesophageal reflux. Take away from mineral supplements, thiamine or alkaloids
Key Constituents	Essential oil (mainly containing menthol and menthone), tannins, flavonoids
Quality or Adulteration Issues	Other species of Mentha may occasionally be present

PHYLLANTHUS

Botanical Names(s)	Phyllanthus amarus
Part Used	Aerial parts
Dose	15 to 40 mL/week (1:2 liquid)
Main Actions	Antiviral, hepatoprotective, hypoglycaemic
Key Indications	Hepatitis, chronic persistent hepatitis, chronic active hepatitis
Other Indications	Type 2 diabetes
Major Safety Issues	None known
Key Constituents	Lignans including phyllanthin, flavonoids, alkaloids, tannins
Quality or Adulteration Issues	Other species of Phyllanthus are potential adulterants

PLEURISY ROOT

Botanical Names(s)	Asclepias tuberosa
Part Used	Root
Dose	10 to 20 mL/week (1:2 liquid)
Main Actions	Diaphoretic, expectorant
Key Indications	Acute bronchitis, pertussis, pleurisy, pneumonia (all acute doses), cough Common cold, influenza, fever (all acute doses)
Major Safety Issues	None known, but see adulteration issues below
Key Constituents	Not well defined

Quality or Adulteration Issues	Commonly adulterated with other species of Asclepias which may contain cardiac glycosides

POKE ROOT

Botanical Names(s)	Phytolacca decandra; P. americana
Part Used	Root
Dose	1 to 5 mL/week (1:5 tincture)
Main Actions	Anti-inflammatory, lymphatic, depurative, immune enhancing
Key Indications	Enlarged lymph glands, lymphadenitis, tonsillitis, pharyngitis, laryngitis, nasopharyngeal catarrh (chronic), mumps Mastitis, mammary abscess Chronic skin disorders, dermatitis Topically for tinea, acne, mastitis
Other Indications	Cancer, especially of the breast or uterus
Major Safety Issues	Use cautiously and do not exceed recommended doses. Contraindicated in pregnancy, lactation, lymphocytic leukaemia, gastrointestinal irritation. Do not apply to broken skin and avoid concurrent use with immunosuppressive drugs
Key Constituents	Triterpenoid saponins (phytolaccosides), sterols, lectins
Quality or Adulteration Issues	No adulterants known

POLYGALA

Botanical Names(s)	Polygala tenuifolia
Part Used	Root bark
Dose	20 to 60 mL/week (1:2 liquid)
Main Actions	Expectorant, sedative

Key Indications	Asthma, acute or chronic bronchitis, bronchiectasis
	Sleep onset insomnia, palpitations, excitability, irritability
Major Safety Issues	Saponins may case or aggravate gastro-oesophageal reflux
Key Constituents	Triterpenoid saponins (including tenuifolin), resin
Quality or Adulteration Issues	No adulterants are documented

POLYGONUM CUSPIDATUM

Botanical Names(s)	Polygonum cuspidatum
Part Used	Rhizome
Dose	7.5 to 30.0 g/day delivering 15 to 60 mg of resveratrol
Main Actions	Antioxidant, anti-inflammatory, antitumour, antiageing
Key Indications	To slow the ageing process
	Prevention of cardiovascular disease
	Osteoarthritis, constipation, leukopaenia, tonsillitis, rheumatoid arthritis
Other Indications	Metabolic syndrome X
Major Safety Issues	No major issues identified
Key Constituents	Resveratrol, piceid, anthraquinones, tannins
Quality or Adulteration Issues	No adulterants known

POLYGONUM MULTIFLORUM

Botanical Names(s)	Polygonum multiflorum
Part Used	Processed root
Dose	50 to 100 mL/week (1:2 liquid)

Main Actions	Nervine tonic, antioxidant, antiageing, hypocholesterolaemic, bitter tonic
Key Indications	To slow the ageing process
	Fatigue with insomnia, debility in the elderly
	To strengthen connective tissue, osteoarthritis
Other Indications	Hypercholesterolaemia
	Tinnitus, dizziness
Major Safety Issues	None known
Key Constituents	Tetrahydroxystilbene glucoside (related to resveratrol), anthraquinones, tannins, phospholipids
Quality or Adulteration Issues	No adulterants known

PRICKLY ASH

Botanical Names(s)	Zanthoxylum clava-herculis; Z. americanum
Part Used	Bark
Dose	10 to 30 mL/week (1:2 liquid)
Main Actions	Circulatory stimulant, diaphoretic, antirheumatic, sialogogue
Key Indications	Impaired peripheral circulation including intermittent claudication, Buerger's disease, Raynaud's syndrome, cerebrovascular disease
	Varicose veins, haemorrhoids
	Leg cramps, osteoarthritis
Other Indications	Rheumatism, neuralgia, restless legs syndrome
Major Safety Issues	None known
Key Constituents	Alkaloids (chelerythrine, nitidine, tembetarine), lignans (asarinin), alkylamides (neoherculin)
Quality or Adulteration Issues	Samples lacking in the characteristic tingling sensation of alkylamides are probably the common adulterant Aralia spinosa

PROPOLIS

Botanical Names(s)	Derived from a number of plant species by bees
Part Used	Resin
Dose	10 to 40 mL/week (1:5 liquid)
Main Actions	Astringent, vulnerary, antibacterial, antifungal, antiparasitic, antiviral, immune modulating, antioxidant, antitumour, local anaesthetic
Key Indications	Common cold, influenza, infectious otitis media, tonsillitis, chronic sinusitis
	Peptic ulcer, gastritis, gastrointestinal infection, mouth ulcers
	Topically for herpes simplex, gingivitis, mouth ulcers, stomatitis, halitosis, wounds, ulcers, burns
Other Indications	Adjunct therapy in cancer
	Ulcerative colitis
Major Safety Issues	Contraindicated in known allergy. Exercise caution in patients with a history of allergy, especially skin rashes
Key Constituents	Constituents vary depending on the area of origin, but good quality propolis contains flavonoids (galangin, pinocembrin etc), phenolic acids and their esters, essential oil
Quality or Adulteration Issues	No adulterants known

QING HAO

Botanical Names(s)	Artemisia annua
Part Used	Herb
Dose	20 to 50 mL/week (1:2 liquid)
Main Actions	Bitter tonic, febrifuge, antiparasitic
Key Indications	Malaria (but not as a preventative), intestinal parasites
	Lupus (high doses)
Major Safety Issues	Best avoided in pregnancy
Key Constituents	Artemisinin (a peroxide-containing sesquiterpene lactone), essential oil, flavonoids
Quality or Adulteration Issues	Commercial products can contain extracts lacking or low in artemisinin

RASPBERRY LEAF

Botanical Names(s)	Rubus idaeus
Part Used	Leaf
Dose	30 to 100 mL/week (1:2 liquid)
	1.2 to 2.4 g/day (tablet)
Main Actions	Astringent, partus preparator, parturifacient, antidiarrhoeal
Key Indications	To prepare for labour (when taken from the second trimester) and to ensure healthy uterine function
	Dysmenorrhoea
	Morning sickness (which extends into the second trimester)
	Mouth ulcers, diarrhoea, stomatitis
	Topically for tonsillitis, conjunctivitis, pharyngitis
Other Indications	Uterine prolapse, uterine haemorrhage, gastrointestinal bleeding
Major Safety Issues	Do not take concurrently with mineral supplements. Best to confine use in pregnancy to the second and third trimesters
Key Constituents	Not well defined. Flavonoids, gallotannins, ellagitannins
Quality or Adulteration Issues	Occasionally raspberry leaf is confused with bramble/ blackberry leaf (Rubus fructicosus)

RED CLOVER FLOWER

Botanical Names(s)	Trifolium pratense
Part Used	Flower
Dose	20 to 40 mL/week (1:2 liquid)
Main Actions	Depurative, antitumour (traditional)
Key Indications	Chronic skin disorders including dermatitis, psoriasis
Other Indications	Adjunct therapy in cancer
Major Safety Issues	No major issues identified for traditional preparations extracted with 25% ethanol
Key Constituents	Isoflavones (including formononetin and biochanin A), flavanols, phenolic acids (including salicylic and p-coumaric acids), essential oil (trace)
Quality or Adulteration Issues	No adulterants known. Only preparations of the tops extracted with a high alcohol percentage contain appreciable levels of isoflavones

REHMANNIA

Botanical Names(s)	Rehmannia glutinosa
Part Used	Uncured root
Dose	30 to 60 mL/week (1:2 liquid) 1.1 to 1.8 g/day (tablet)
Main Actions	Antipyretic, adrenal tonic, antihaemorrhagic, anti-inflammatory
Key Indications	Adrenal depletion, autoimmune disease Rheumatoid arthritis, asthma, urticaria Chronic nephritis (with Astragalus) Fever, constipation, haematuria, metrorrhagia, epistaxis
Other Indications	Osteoarthritis To support withdrawal from corticosteroid drugs
Major Safety Issues	No major issues identified but caution in pregnancy
Key Constituents	Iridoid glycosides (aucubin, catalpol), rehmanniosides A to D, phenethylalcohol glycosides, jioglutosides, rehmaglutins A to D
Quality or Adulteration Issues	No issues identified

REISHI

Botanical Names(s)	Ganoderma lucidum
Part Used	Mushroom
Dose	20 to 27 g/day (tablet)
Main Actions	Tonic, immune modulating
Key Indications	Adjunct therapy in cancer During chemotherapy or radiotherapy for cancer Chronic infections, chronic immune deficiency To slow ageing, as a tonic for the elderly, convalescence
Other Indications	HIV/AIDS Autoimmune disease Post-viral syndromes, chronic fatigue syndrome, fibromyalgia
Major Safety Issues	No major issues identified
Key Constituents	Polysaccharides, triterpene acids
Quality or Adulteration Issues	Other species of Ganoderma can be adulterants

RHODIOLA

Botanical Names(s)	Rhodiola rosea
Part Used	Root
Dose	20 to 40 mL/week (2:1 liquid) 6 to 12 g/day (tablet)

Main Actions	Adaptogenic, tonic, antioxidant, antitumour
Key Indications	Debility, emaciation, cachexia, chronic immune deficiency
	Fatigue, physical stress, convalescence, failure to thrive
	During chemotherapy or radiotherapy for cancer
	To improve physical performance, impotence
	As a tonic for the elderly
	To improve mental performance, concentration and memory, especially when under stress
	Chronic fatigue syndrome, fibromyalgia, post-viral syndromes
Other Indications	HIV/AIDS (as adjunctive treatment)
Major Safety Issues	Take away from mineral supplements. Concurrent use with stimulants is best avoided
Key Constituents	Phenylpropanoids (collectively known as rosavins including rosavin, rosarin, rosin), salidroside, rosiridin, flavonoids, tannins, essential oil (trace)
Quality or Adulteration Issues	Can be substituted with other species of Rhodiola which are lacking rosavins

RHUBARB ROOT

Botanical Names(s)	Rheum palmatum
Part Used	Root and rhizome
Dose	10 to 30 mL/week (1:2 liquid)
Main Actions	Laxative, styptic, antipyretic, antibacterial, anti-inflammatory, antiuraemic
Key Indications	Constipation, gastrointestinal bleeding, dysentery
	Hypercholesterolaemia, elevated triglycerides
	Peptic ulcer to treat Helicobacter
Other Indications	Nephritis, mild renal failure
	Acute pancreatitis
	Endometriosis
Major Safety Issues	Laxative doses (higher doses) for short-term use only. Caution with laxative doses in irritable bowel syndrome, pregnancy, lactation and gastrointestinal inflammation. Caution in children. Take away from mineral supplements.
Key Constituents	Anthraquinone glycosides, phenolics, tannins
Quality or Adulteration Issues	Other species of Rheum are potential adulterants

RIBWORT

Botanical Names(s)	Plantago lanceolata
Part Used	Leaf
Dose	20 to 40 mL/week (1:2 liquid)
Main Actions	Anticatarrhal, demulcent, astringent, vulnerary, styptic
Key Indications	Nasopharyngeal catarrh, chronic sinusitis, hay fever, serous otitis media, pharyngitis, catarrhal deafness, sinus headache
	Lower respiratory catarrh, chronic bronchitis, bronchiectasis, cough
	Peptic ulcer, gastritis
	Topically for leg ulcers, varicose ulcers, pharyngitis, laryngitis
Major Safety Issues	None known
Key Constituents	Iridoids, mucilage, zinc (reputedly), tannins
Quality or Adulteration Issues	No adulterants known

ROSEHIPS

Botanical Names(s)	Rosa canina
Part Used	Fruit
Dose	20 to 40 mL/week (1:5 liquid)
Main Actions	Anti-inflammatory, astringent
Key Indications	Osteoarthritis (higher doses)
	Vitamin C deficiency
	Gastritis, diarrhoea
Major Safety Issues	None known
Key Constituents	Ascorbic acid, fruit acids, flavonoids, mucilage, tannin, carotenoids
Quality or Adulteration Issues	No adulterants known

ROSEMARY

Botanical Names(s)	Rosmarinus officinalis
Part Used	Leaf
Dose	15 to 30 mL/week (1:2 liquid)
	1.5 to 3.0 g/day (tablet)
Main Actions	Carminative, spasmolytic, antioxidant, antimicrobial, circulatory stimulant, hepatoprotective
Key Indications	To improve memory, concentration or mental performance
	To enhance phase II liver detoxification
	Prevention of cardiovascular disease
	Tension headache, debility
	Topically for myalgia, sciatica, neuralgia, wound healing, hair loss
Other Indications	Alzheimer's disease, Parkinson's disease (cerebral antioxidant)
	ADHD
	To slow the ageing process
Major Safety Issues	Take away from mineral supplements
Key Constituents	Essential oil (cineole, alpha-pinene, camphor), phenolic diterpenes (carnosol, carnosic acid), rosmarinic acids, flavonoids, triterpenoids
Quality or Adulteration Issues	Adulteration is uncommon

SAGE

Botanical Names(s)	Salvia officinalis, S. triloba
Part Used	Aerial parts
Dose	15 to 30 mL/week (1:2 liquid)
	0.9 to 1.8 g/day (tablet)
Main Actions	Spasmolytic, antioxidant, astringent, antihyperhidrotic, antimicrobial
Key Indications	Menopausal symptoms, excessive sweating
	To improve memory and concentration
	Dyspepsia, flatulence
	To inhibit lactation
	Topically for laryngitis, pharyngitis, gingivitis, stomatitis, tonsillitis, glossitis
Other Indications	Alzheimer's disease
	Fatigue, tension headache, fever
Major Safety Issues	Contraindicated in pregnancy and lactation (except to stop milk flow). Caution with long-term use (except for low thujone varieties)
Key Constituents	Essential oil, up to 2.5%, containing monoterpenoids such as alpha- and beta-thujone, camphor and cineole. Diterpenoids such as carnosic acid and carnosol, triterpenoids, flavonoids such as 5-methoxysalvigenin, phenolic acids
Quality or Adulteration Issues	Occasional substitution by other species of Salvia

SARSAPARILLA

Botanical Names(s)	Smilax ornata; S. aristolochiaefolia; S. regelii; S. febrifuga; S. medica
Part Used	Root and rhizome
Dose	20 to 40 mL/week (1:2 liquid) 1.2 to 2.4 g/day (tablet)
Main Actions	Depurative, anti-inflammatory, antirheumatic
Key Indications	Chronic skin disorders, especially psoriasis, dermatitis Rheumatoid arthritis, gout, nephritis, rheumatism Debility, fatigue, physical stress
Other Indications	Reputedly a male tonic (and does contain saponins with some similarity to Tribulus), however is not a source of testosterone as claimed by some
Major Safety Issues	Saponins can cause or aggravate gastro-oesophageal reflux
Key Constituents	The complexity of the various Smilax species used means that key constituents have not been conclusively determined. Steroidal saponins (including parillin), phytosterols, resin
Quality or Adulteration Issues	Other species of Smilax to those listed above are known adulterants

SAW PALMETTO

Botanical Names(s)	Serenoa repens; Sabal serrulata
Part Used	Fruit
Dose	20 to 60 mL/week (1:2 liquid) 2.2 to 3.2 g/day (capsule)
Main Actions	Anti-inflammatory, male tonic, antiprostatic, spasmolytic, possibly antiandrogenic
Key Indications	Benign prostatic hyperplasia, chronic prostatitis Inflammation of the genitourinary tract including orchitis, cystitis, salpingitis, pelvic inflammatory disease Male and female infertility
Other Indications	Underdeveloped mammary glands, male impotence, testicular atrophy
Major Safety Issues	Caution with concurrent use of warfarin
Key Constituents	Free fatty acids, triglycerides, phytosterols (mainly beta-sitosterol), flavonoids, polysaccharides
Quality or Adulteration Issues	No adulterants known

SCHISANDRA

Botanical Names(s)	Schisandra chinensis
Part Used	Fruit
Dose	25 to 60 mL/week (1:2 liquid) 3.0 to 5.0 g/day (tablet)
Main Actions	Hepatoprotective, antioxidant, adaptogenic, nervine tonic, antitussive, oxytocic, mild antidepressant
Key Indications	To enhance phase I/II detoxification by the liver, chronic hepatitis, chronic liver damage Fatigue, physical stress, debility To improve physical, exercise and mental performance and concentration
Other Indications	Night sweats, enuresis nocturia
Major Safety Issues	Traditionally contraindicated in pregnancy except to assist childbirth. May enhance the clearance of prescribed drugs (theoretical concern)

Key Constituents	Dibenzocyclooctene lignans (about 2% by weight), such as schisandrin, schisandrins A to C and gomisin A, essential oil (about 3%)
Quality or Adulteration Issues	Other species of Schisandra are the most common adulterants

SENNA PODS

Botanical Names(s)	Cassia senna; Cassia angustifolia
Part Used	Fruit
Dose	10 to 40 mL/week (1:2 liquid)
Main Actions	Laxative
Key Indications	Constipation
	Haemorrhoids or anal fissure (to soften the stool, cathartic doses to be avoided)
Major Safety Issues	For short-term use only. Caution in pregnancy, lactation, irritable bowel syndrome and gastrointestinal inflammation. Caution in children. Contraindicated in diarrhoea or with digoxin
Key Constituents	Anthraquinone glycosides (sennosides A and B)
Quality or Adulteration Issues	No adulterants known

SHATAVARI

Botanical Names(s)	Asparagus racemosus
Part Used	Root
Dose	30 to 60 mL/week (1:2 liquid)
	1.2 to 2.4 g/day (tablet)
Main Actions	Tonic, galactagogue, sexual tonic, adaptogenic, spasmolytic, antidiarrhoeal, diuretic

Key Indications	Menopausal symptoms
	Infertility or low libido in women (especially) and men, male impotence
	To promote lactation, sexual debility
Major Safety Issues	Saponins may cause or aggravate gastro-oesophageal reflux
Key Constituents	Steroidal saponins, including shatavarin-l, alkaloids, including the nontoxic pyrrolizidine alkaloid asparagamine A, mucilage
Quality or Adulteration Issues	No adulterants known

SHEEP SORREL

Botanical Names(s)	Rumex acetosella
Part Used	Aerial parts
Dose	400 to 600 mg/day (tablet)
Main Actions	Immune modulating, antitumour (traditional)
Key Indications	As part of a traditional formulation for:
	Adjunctive treatment of cancer
	During chemotherapy or radiotherapy for cancer
Other Indications	Poor immunity, HIV/AIDS
Major Safety Issues	Avoid excessive doses in renal disease due to the oxalate content
Key Constituents	Not well defined. Flavonoids, oxalate, organic acids
Quality or Adulteration Issues	Can be adulterated with sorrel (Rumex acetosa)

SHEPHERD'S PURSE

Botanical Names(s)	Capsella bursa-pastoris
Part Used	Aerial parts
Dose	20 to 40 mL/week (1:2 liquid) 1.9 to 2.6 g/day (tablet)
Main Actions	Antihaemorrhagic, uterine antihaemorrhagic, urinary antiseptic, styptic
Key Indications	Menorrhagia (acute doses may be necessary), metrorrhagia Dysfunctional uterine bleeding Acute cystitis, haematuria (all acute doses) Topically for epistaxis, uterine haemorrhage, menorrhagia
Major Safety Issues	Caution in pregnancy and lactation
Key Constituents	Not well defined. Glucosinolates, flavonoids, amino acids, organic acids, essential oil (trace), amines
Quality or Adulteration Issues	No adulterants known

SHIITAKE

Botanical Names(s)	Lentinula edodes
Part Used	Mushroom
Dose	2.4 to 4.0 g/day (tablet)
Main Actions	Immune modulating, antitumour
Key Indications	Adjunct therapy in cancer During chemotherapy or radiotherapy for cancer Chronic infections, chronic immune deficiency
Other Indications	HIV/AIDS Autoimmune disease
	Post-viral syndromes, chronic fatigue syndrome, fibromyalgia
Major Safety Issues	Contraindicated in known allergy
Key Constituents	Polysaccharides (especially lentinan)
Quality or Adulteration Issues	No adulterants known

SIBERIAN GINSENG (ELEUTHEROCOCCUS)

Botanical Names(s)	Eleutherococcus senticosus; Acanthopanax senticosus
Part Used	Root
Dose	15 to 55 mL/week (1:2 liquid) 2.5 to 6.3 g/day (tablet)
Main Actions	Adaptogenic, immune modulating
Key Indications	Physical stress, fatigue, convalescence, mild depression Cancer during chemotherapy and especially radiotherapy To improve physical, exercise and mental performance and concentration Debility, chronic immune deficiency, as a tonic for the elderly
Other Indications	Post-viral syndromes, chronic fatigue syndrome, fibromyalgia
Major Safety Issues	Best avoided during acute phases of infections
Key Constituents	Eleutherosides (a chemically diverse group of compounds), especially eleutheroside E. Minor constituents are triterpenoid saponins and glycans
Quality or Adulteration Issues	Periploca sepium is recorded as a substitute for Siberian ginseng. Products should be standardised for eleutheroside E.

SKULLCAP

Botanical Names(s)	Scutellaria lateriflora
Part Used	Aerial parts
Dose	15 to 30 mL/week (1:2 liquid) 1.5 to 2.0 g/day (tablet)
Main Actions	Nervine tonic, mild sedative, spasmolytic
Key Indications	Excitability, irritability, emotional stress, anxiety, epilepsy, premenstrual syndrome Insomnia (especially sleep maintenance), nervous fatigue
Other Indications	Tension headache, depression, neuralgia
Major Safety Issues	No major issues identified. Attribution of hepatotoxic effects most likely applies to adulterants (see below)
Key Constituents	Flavonoids (baicalin, scutellarin), diterpenes (low levels, structures disputed), amino acids, essential oil (trace), caffeic acid
Quality or Adulteration Issues	This herb is frequently adulterated with other species of Scutellaria or Teucrium species

SLIPPERY ELM

Botanical Names(s)	Ulmus rubra; U. fulva
Part Used	Inner stem bark
Dose	1.6 to 4.0 g/day (capsule)
Main Actions	Demulcent, emollient, laxative
Key Indications	Gastritis, peptic ulcer (take before meals), gastro-oesophageal reflux (take after meals and before bed) Ulcerative colitis, irritable bowel syndrome, constipation, diverticulosis, gastrointestinal inflammation
	Haemorrhoids or anal fissure (to soften the stool, higher doses required) To modify bowel flora
Major Safety Issues	Take with plenty of water. Contraindicated in intestinal obstruction. Take at least 2 hours away from prescribed drugs
Key Constituents	Mucilage, starch, tannins (small amount)
Quality or Adulteration Issues	Can be adulterated with the outer bark. (Only the inner bark contains the necessary level of mucilage). Alcoholic extracts and tinctures are inactive due to the insolubility of mucilage in alcohol

SQUAW VINE

Botanical Names(s)	Mitchella repens
Part Used	Whole plant
Dose	20 to 40 mL/week (1:2 liquid)
Main Actions	Partus preparator, parturifacient, astringent, spasmolytic
Key Indications	To prepare for and facilitate labour Spasmodic dysmenorrhoea
Other Indications	History of threatened miscarriage (was used throughout the entire pregnancy)
Major Safety Issues	Generally used later in pregnancy from the sixth month onwards
Key Constituents	Not well defined. Saponins, tannins
Quality or Adulteration Issues	No adulterants known

STEMONA

Botanical Names(s)	Stemona japonica; S. sessifolia; S. tuberosa
Part Used	Root
Dose	3 to 6 g/day (tablet)

Main Actions	Anthelmintic, antifungal, antitussive
Key Indications	Intestinal worms Cough
Other Indications	Topically for fungal, lice or scabies infestation
Major Safety Issues	No major issues identified
Key Constituents	Alkaloids including stemonine and tuberostemonine
Quality or Adulteration Issues	No adulterants known

ST JOHN'S WORT

Botanical Names(s)	Hypericum perforatum
Part Used	Aerial parts
Dose	15 to 40 mL/week (1:2 liquid) 3.6 to 7.2 g/day (tablet)
Main Actions	Antidepressant, nervine tonic, antiviral, vulnerary, antimicrobial (topically)
Key Indications	Depression, anxiety, irritability, emotional stress Menopausal symptoms, premenstrual syndrome Herpes simplex, hepatitis, shingles, viral infections (enveloped viruses) Neuralgia, sciatica, trigeminal neuralgia Insomnia (sleep onset or sleep maintenance)
Other Indications	Autoimmune disease
Major Safety Issues	Not to be solely relied on in severe depression. High hyperforin preparations (such as tablets) are contraindicated with the following drugs: verapamil, irinotecan, imatinib, HIV drugs, cyclosporin, methadone, anticoagulants, digoxin and the oral contraceptive pill. Caution with all other drugs. Avoid excessive exposure to sunlight
Key Constituents	Hypericin, pseudohypericin, hyperforin, flavonoids, procyanidins, essential oil
Quality or Adulteration Issues	Commercial crude herb raw material can contain subtherapeutic quantities of hypericin

ST MARY'S THISTLE (MILK THISTLE)

Botanical Names(s)	Silybum marianum
Part Used	Seed
Dose	30 to 60 mL/week (1:1 liquid) 30 to 60 g/day (tablet) containing 280 to 560 mg flavanolignans
Main Actions	Hepatoprotective, hepatic trophorestorative, antioxidant, choleretic
Key Indications	Liver damage, liver cirrhosis, hepatitis A, B and C, fatty liver, chronic active hepatitis Gall stones, digestive liver insufficiency, dyspepsia Nausea, flatulent colic, constipation, flatulence, abdominal bloating Type 2 diabetes, metabolic syndrome X Haemochromatosis, to reduce heavy metal burden
Other Indications	Food allergies/sensitivities During chemotherapy for cancer, to reduce anaesthesia toxicity
Major Safety Issues	Contraindicated in known allergy
Key Constituents	Flavanolignans (collectively known as silymarin) including silybin, silychristin, silydianin
Quality or Adulteration Issues	Liquid preparations will be devoid of silymarin unless they contain at least 45% ethanol

SUNDEW

Botanical Names(s)	Drosera longifolia
Part Used	Aerial parts
Dose	10 to 20 mL/week (1:5 liquid)
Main Actions	Spasmolytic, demulcent, expectorant
Key Indications	Acute bronchitis, pertussis, tracheitis Chronic bronchitis, asthma
Other Indications	Gastritis, peptic ulcer
Major Safety Issues	None known
Key Constituents	Not well defined. Naphthoquinones including plumbagin
Quality or Adulteration Issues	Drosera rotundifolia is protected due to its critically endangered status and should not be used

TERMINALIA ARJUNA

Botanical Names(s)	Terminalia arjuna
Part Used	Bark
Dose	20 to 40 mL/week (1:2 liquid)
Main Actions	Cardioprotective, hypocholesterolaemic, mild diuretic, hepatoprotective
Key Indications	Angina pectoris, to prevent heart attacks, cardiomyopathy Mild congestive cardiac failure, cardiac arrhythmias
Other Indications	Hypercholesterolaemia
Major Safety Issues	No major issues identified
Key Constituents	Triterpenoid saponins (arjunglucosides), flavonoids (arjunone, arjunolone), phytosterols, tannins
Quality or Adulteration Issues	No adulterants known

THUJA

Botanical Names(s)	Thuja occidentalis
Part Used	Leaf
Dose	15 to 30 mL/week (1:5 liquid) 400 to 800 mg/day (tablet)
Main Actions	Antimicrobial, depurative, antiviral, antifungal
Key Indications	Warts (also topically), viral infections Common cold, acute sinusitis Topically for warts, fungal infections
Other Indications	Adjunct therapy in cancer (controversial)
Major Safety Issues	Contraindicated in pregnancy and lactation. Do not exceed recommended doses. Best avoided with epilepsy
Key Constituents	Essential oil (mainly thujone), resin, podophyllotoxins
Quality or Adulteration Issues	Other species of Thuja are likely adulterants due to their botanical similarity

THYME

Botanical Names(s)	Thymus vulgaris
Part Used	Leaf and flower
Dose	15 to 40 mL/week (1:2 liquid) 40 to 60 mg/day (essential oil)
Main Actions	Expectorant, spasmolytic, antibacterial, antifungal, antioxidant, rubefacient (topically), antimicrobial
Key Indications	Acute bronchitis, whooping cough, nasopharyngeal catarrh, pharyngitis, laryngitis, common cold, pertussis Chronic bronchitis, bronchiectasis, bronchial asthma, cough Dyspepsia, chronic gastritis, diarrhoea

	Topically for tonsillitis, pharyngitis, stomatitis, gingivitis, halitosis
Other Indications	Peptic ulcer for Helicobacter Enuresis nocturia
Major Safety Issues	Avoid in known allergy
Key Constituents	Essential oil containing mainly phenols (thymol, carvacrol), carnosol, carnosic acid, biphenyls, flavonoids, phenolic acids, acetophenone glycosides
Quality or Adulteration Issues	There are several subspecies of Thymus vulgaris which should be avoided due to their low phenol content

TIENCHI GINSENG

Botanical Names(s)	Panax notoginseng
Part Used	Root
Dose	25 to 60 mL/week (1:2 liquid)
Main Actions	Antihaemorrhagic, cardioprotective, anti-inflammatory, antiarrhythmic, hypocholesterolaemic
Key Indications	Menorrhagia, metrorrhagia, uterine haemorrhage Haemoptysis, haematuria, gastrointestinal bleeding Traumatic injury especially with haematoma and bruising Angina pectoris, cardiac arrhythmias, hypercholesterolaemia
Other Indications	To assist with weight loss
Major Safety Issues	Traditionally contraindicated in pregnancy
Key Constituents	Ginsenosides (in differing relative amounts to Panax ginseng)
Quality or Adulteration Issues	No adulterants known

TRIBULUS LEAF

Botanical Names(s)	Tribulus terrestris
Part Used	Aerial parts
Dose	50 to 100 mL/week (2:1 liquid) Standardised extract doses delivering 200 to 400 mg/day furostanol saponins (as a tablet)
Main Actions	Tonic, aphrodisiac, oestrogenic in females (indirectly), androgenic in males (indirectly), fertility agent
Key Indications	Male infertility, impotence, decreased libido Female infertility, menopausal symptoms, polycystic ovary syndrome To improve physical or exercise performance Fatigue, convalescence, physical stress
Major Safety Issues	Saponins can cause or aggravate gastro-oesophageal reflux. Caution in patients with pre-existing cholestasis
Key Constituents	Steroidal saponins (including protodioscin, protogracillin), phytosterols. The presence of harmala alkaloids is disputed
Quality or Adulteration Issues	The root or fruit are often substitutes for the leaf in modern products, but are unlikely to have the same therapeutic profile. Analysis for furostanol saponins should be by HPLC

TRUE UNICORN

Botanical Names(s)	Aletris farinosa
Part Used	Root
Dose	12 to 40 mL/week (1:2 liquid)
Main Actions	Bitter, spasmolytic, mild sedative, uterine tonic
Key Indications	Anorexia, dyspepsia Threatened miscarriage, female infertility, uterine weakness

According to King's Dispensatory the female uses are disputed and possibly based on confusion with False Unicorn

Major Safety Issues	None known
Key Constituents	Not well defined
Quality or Adulteration Issues	No adulterants known

TURMERIC

Botanical Names(s)	Curcuma longa
Part Used	Rhizome
Dose	35 to 100 mL/week (1:1 liquid) 4.0 to 10.0 g/day (tablet)
Main Actions	Anti-inflammatory, antiplatelet, antioxidant, hypolipidaemic, choleretic
Key Indications	Peptic ulcer (including for Helicobacter), dyspepsia Osteoarthritis, rheumatoid arthritis To enhance phase I/II detoxification by the liver Asthma Topically for chronic skin disorders
Other Indications	To prevent cancer, Alzheimer's disease and cardiovascular disease Cystic fibrosis Hypercholesterolaemia
Major Safety Issues	Caution with high doses in patients taking antiplatelet or anticoagulant drugs
Key Constituents	Essential oil, curcuminoids (mainly curcumin)
Quality or Adulteration Issues	Other species of Curcuma are possible adulterants

TYLOPHORA

Botanical Names(s)	Tylophora indica
Part Used	Leaf
Dose	5 to 15 mL/week (1:5 liquid) for the first 10 to 14 days of each month (dispense separately from other liquid herbs)
Main Actions	Antiasthmatic, anti-inflammatory, immune depressant, antiallergic, emetic
Key Indications	Asthma, hay fever Autoimmune disease, lupus, rheumatoid arthritis, multiple sclerosis
Major Safety Issues	Contraindicated in pregnancy and lactation and for long-term use. Can cause nausea and vomiting at normal therapeutic doses, start with 10 to 20 drops per day and build up to a maximum tolerated dose within the recommended range (see above)
Key Constituents	Alkaloids including tylophorine, tylophorinine
Quality or Adulteration Issues	No adulterants known

VALERIAN

Botanical Names(s)	Valeriana officinalis
Part Used	Root and rhizome
Dose	15 to 40 mL/week (1:2 liquid) 2.1 to 3.5 g/day (tablet)
Main Actions	Anxiolytic, mild sedative, hypnotic, spasmolytic
Key Indications	Anxiety, excitability, panic attacks, emotional stress, irritability Insomnia (sleep onset or maintenance) Nervous dyspepsia, intestinal colic Hypertension, tension headache

Other Indications	Depression, migraine headache, dysmenorrhoea
Major Safety Issues	No major issues identified
Key Constituents	Valepotriates, essential oil, valerenic acid and derivatives
Quality or Adulteration Issues	Other species of Valeriana are known adulterants

VERVAIN

Botanical Names(s)	Verbena officinalis
Part Used	Aerial parts
Dose	20 to 40 mL/week (1:2 liquid)
Main Actions	Nervine tonic, thymoleptic, diaphoretic astringent, galactagogue
Key Indications	Anorexia, infantile colic
	Influenza, fever
	Insufficient lactation
	Anxiety, irritability, mild depression
Major Safety Issues	Take away from mineral supplements
Key Constituents	Iridoid glycosides (verbenalin, aucubin), hydroxycinnamic acid derivatives (verbascoside), flavonoids, triterpenes, sterols
Quality or Adulteration Issues	May be adulterated with other species of Verbena

VIOLET LEAF

Botanical Names(s)	Viola odorata
Part Used	Leaf
Dose	12 to 25 mL/week (1:2 liquid)
Main Actions	Expectorant, antitumour (reputed), demulcent, diaphoretic
Key Indications	Chronic bronchitis, cough, asthma
	Chronic nasopharyngeal catarrh, common cold

Other Indications	Adjunctive treatment in cancer
Major Safety Issues	None known
Key Constituents	Not well defined. Essential oil (trace), flavonoids, saponins, salicylates, macrocyclic peptides, phenolic acids
Quality or Adulteration Issues	Other species of Viola are potential adulterants

WHITE HOREHOUND

Botanical Names(s)	Marrubium vulgare
Part Used	Aerial parts
Dose	15 to 40 mL/week (1:2 liquid)
	0.6 to 1.2 g/day (tablet)
Main Actions	Expectorant, spasmolytic, bitter tonic
Key Indications	Acute bronchitis, common cold (acute doses for both), pertussis
	Asthma, chronic bronchitis
	Dyspepsia, flatulence, anorexia
Major Safety Issues	No major issues identified
Key Constituents	Diterpene lactones and alcohols (marrubiin, marrubiol), flavonoids, alkaloids (betonicine), essential oil (trace)
Quality or Adulteration Issues	White horehound has been adulterated with other Marrubium spp. Black horehound (Ballota nigra) as well as Ballota hirsuta have been adulterants

WILD CHERRY

Botanical Names(s)	Prunus serotina
Part Used	Bark
Dose	15 to 30 mL/week (1:2 liquid)
Main Actions	Antitussive, mild sedative, astringent

Key Indications	Cough, bronchitis, tracheitis, pleurisy, pneumonia, pertussis
	Common cold
Major Safety Issues	Long-term use is best avoided
Key Constituents	Cyanogenic glycoside (prunasin), phenolic acids, tannins
Quality or Adulteration Issues	Barks from other species of Prunus can be substituted

WILD YAM

Botanical Names(s)	Dioscorea villosa
Part Used	Root and rhizome
Dose	20 to 40 mL/week (1:2 liquid)
	1.2 to 2.4 g/day (tablet)
Main Actions	Spasmolytic, anti-inflammatory, antirheumatic, oestrogen-modulating
Key Indications	Menopausal symptoms (oral use only)
	Spasmodic dysmenorrhoea, intestinal colic, diverticulitis, ovarian pain
	Female infertility, threatened miscarriage
	The value of wild yam creams for topical use for menopausal symptoms is questionable
Other Indications	Rheumatoid arthritis
Major Safety Issues	Saponins may cause or aggravate gastro-oesophageal reflux
Key Constituents	Steroidal saponins (major one resembles but is not dioscin). Only contains diosgenin as glycosidic derivatives (saponins)
Quality or Adulteration Issues	Other species of Dioscorea and commercial extracts for the chemical industry (largely containing free diosgenin) are common adulterants

WILLOW BARK

Botanical Names(s)	Salix alba; S. daphnoides; S. purpurea; S. fragilis
Part Used	Bark
Dose	25 to 50 mL/week (1:2 liquid)
	16 to 24 g/day (tablet)
Main Actions	Anti-inflammatory, analgesic, antirheumatic, antipyretic
Key Indications	Osteoarthritis, rheumatoid arthritis, low back pain, ankylosing spondylitis
	Fever, migraine headache, tension headache
	Generally the use of willow bark in tablet form is recommended as it is clinically proven and delivers higher doses
Major Safety Issues	Contraindicated in known allergy to salicylates and glucose-6-phosphate dehydrogenase deficiency. Best avoided in breastfeeding. Use cautiously in conjunction with anticoagulant and antiplatelet drugs
Key Constituents	Phenolic glycosides (2.5% to 11%, such as salicin and salicin esters), flavonoids, condensed tannins (8% to 20%)
Quality or Adulteration Issues	No adulterants known. However, the level of salicin should be quantified

WILLOW HERB

Botanical Names(s)	Epilobium parviflorum
Part Used	Aerial parts
Dose	20 to 40 mL/week (1:2 liquid)
Main Actions	Antiprostatic
Key Indications	Benign prostatic hyperplasia
	Prostate cancer (adjunct therapy)
Major Safety Issues	Take away from mineral supplements

Key Constituents	Not well defined. Hydrolysable tannins (including the ellagitannin oenothein B), flavonoids (especially myricitrin), triterpenes, sterols
Quality or Adulteration Issues	While the smaller-growing Epilobium species are acceptable substitutes, the larger ones such as E. angustifolium are unacceptable

WITCH HAZEL LEAF

Botanical Names(s)	Hamamelis virginiana
Part Used	Leaf
Dose	20 to 40 mL/week (1:2 liquid)
Main Actions	Astringent, anti-inflammatory, styptic
Key Indications	Diarrhoea, gastrointestinal bleeding
	Topically for haemorrhoids, wounds, dermatitis, chronic skin disorders, menorrhagia, varicose veins
Major Safety Issues	Avoid topical use in known allergy. Take away from mineral supplements
Key Constituents	Condensed and hydrolysable tannins (hamamelitannin, procyanidins, gallotannins), essential oil, flavonoids, phenolic acids
Quality or Adulteration Issues	No adulterants known

WITHANIA (ASHWAGANDA)

Botanical Names(s)	Withania somnifera
Part Used	Root
Dose	20 to 50 mL/week (1:1 liquid)
	2.9 to 4.8 g/day (tablet)
Main Actions	Tonic, adaptogenic, mild sedative, anti-inflammatory, immune modulating, antianaemic
Key Indications	Debility, emaciation, cachexia, anaemia, chronic immune deficiency, leukopaenia
	Fatigue, physical stress, convalescence, failure to thrive
	During chemotherapy or radiotherapy for cancer
	To improve physical performance, impotence
	As a tonic for the elderly
	Insomnia, osteoarthritis
	Chronic fatigue syndrome, fibromyalgia, post-viral syndromes
Other Indications	HIV/AIDS (as adjunctive treatment)
	Drug abuse or addiction
Major Safety Issues	No major issues identified
Key Constituents	Steroidal compounds (withanolides) including withaferin A and sitoindosides, tropane-type alkaloids
Quality or Adulteration Issues	Some varieties (and other species) of Withania are very low in withanolides

WOOD BETONY

Botanical Names(s)	Stachys betonica
Part Used	Aerial parts
Dose	15 to 30 mL/week (1:2 liquid)
Main Actions	Sedative, bitter tonic
Key Indications	Tension headache, dizziness, anxiety, neuralgia
Other Indications	Menière's disease
Major Safety Issues	None known
Key Constituents	Not well defined. Alkaloids including betonicine and stachydrine
Quality or Adulteration Issues	No adulterants known

WORMWOOD

Botanical Names(s)	Artemisia absinthium
Part Used	Aerial parts
Dose	5 to 20 mL/week (1:5 liquid)
	300 to 600 mg/day (tablet)
Main Actions	Bitter tonic, anthelmintic, antiparasitic
Key Indications	Intestinal worms, intestinal parasites
	Digestive weakness, hypochlorhydria, anorexia
	Flatulence, flatulent colic, intestinal colic, abdominal bloating, nausea
	Food allergies/sensitivities
	Crohn's disease, autoimmune disease
Other Indications	Common cold, influenza
Major Safety Issues	Contraindicated in pregnancy and lactation and in known allergy. Excessive doses will cause headaches. Caution in peptic ulcer disease and hyperacidity
Key Constituents	Intensely bitter sesquiterpene lactone dimers (absinthin, artabsinthin), essential oil (mainly thujone), phenolic acids, flavonols
Quality or Adulteration Issues	Occasionally adulterated with Artemisia vulgaris

YARROW

Botanical Names(s)	Achillea millefolium
Part Used	Aerial parts
Dose	15 to 40 mL/week (1:2 liquid)
	1.0 to 2.0 g/day (tablet)
Main Actions	Diaphoretic, antipyretic, peripheral vasodilator, anti-inflammatory, spasmolytic, bitter tonic, styptic (haemostatic), antimicrobial, antihaemorrhagic, vulnerary
Key Indications	Menorrhagia, gastrointestinal bleeding
	Common cold, influenza, fever (all acute doses)
	Anorexia, dyspepsia, intestinal colic
	Topically for dermatitis, chronic skin disorders
Other Indications	Hypertension
Major Safety Issues	Contraindicated in known allergy
Key Constituents	Essential oil, sesquiterpene lactones, flavonoids, alkaloids, betonicine, polyacetylenes, phenolic acids
Quality or Adulteration Issues	Other species and chemotypes of Achillea are known adulterants

YELLOW DOCK

Botanical Names(s)	Rumex crispus
Part Used	Root
Dose	15 to 30 mL/week (1:2 liquid)
	0.8 to 2.0 g/day (tablet)
Main Actions	Mild laxative, cholagogue, depurative
Key Indications	Dermatitis, psoriasis, chronic skin disorders
	Constipation
Other Indications	Rheumatism, osteoarthritis, rheumatoid arthritis
Major Safety Issues	Avoid excessively laxative doses, especially in ileus (intestinal obstruction)
Key Constituents	Anthraquinone glycosides
Quality or Adulteration Issues	No adulterants known

ZIZYPHUS (SPINY JUJUBE)

Botanical Names(s)	Zizyphus spinosa
Part Used	Seed
Dose	40 to 80 mL/week (1:2 liquid)
	2.7 to 4.5 g/day (tablet)
Main Actions	Hypnotic, mild sedative, hypotensive, anxiolytic
Key Indications	Anxiety (especially with excessive sweating), insomnia (sleep onset), emotional stress
	Night sweats, irritability, palpitations
Other Indications	Hypertension
Major Safety Issues	Caution in patients with severe diarrhoea
Key Constituents	Dammarane-type saponins (0.2%), known as jujubosides A and B, and a flavone C-glycoside called spinosin
Quality or Adulteration Issues	No adulterants known

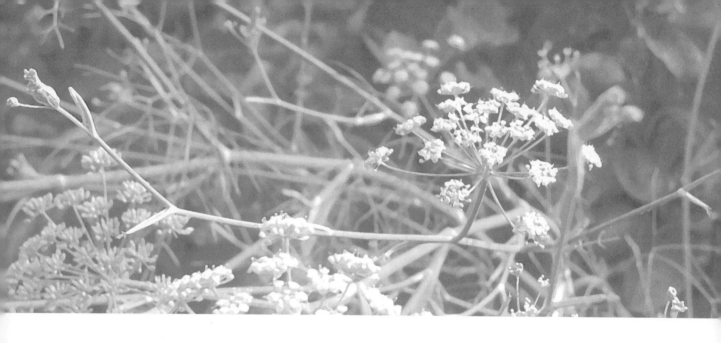

Actions Index

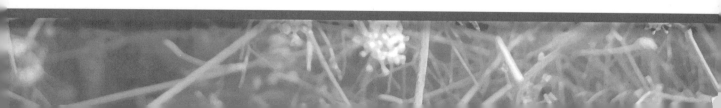

ADAPTOGENIC

Astragalus, Siberian Ginseng, Gotu Kola, Korean Ginseng, Rhodiola, Schisandra, Shatavari, Withania

ADRENAL TONIC

Licorice, Rehmannia

ANALGESIC

Arnica (topically only), California Poppy, Cloves, Corydalis, Devil's Claw, Jamaica Dogwood, Kava (mild), Pasque Flower, Peppermint (topically), Willow Bark

ANAPHRODISIAC

Hops

ANTACID

Meadowsweet

ANTHELMINTIC

Andrographis, Black Walnut, Cloves, Feverfew, Garlic, Mugwort, Myrrh, Stemona, Wormwood

ANTIAGEING

Polygonum cuspidatum, Polygonum multiflorum

ANTIALLERGIC

Albizia, Baical Skullcap, Evening Primrose Oil, Feverfew, Paeonia, Nettle Leaf, Tylophora

ANTIANAEMIC

Withania, Dong Quai

ANTIANDROGENIC

Hops, Saw Palmetto (possibly)

ANTIARRHYTHMIC

Corydalis, Dong Quai, Hawthorn (leaf & berry), Motherwort, Tienchi Ginseng

ANTIASTHMATIC

Black Haw, Tylophora

ANTIBACTERIAL

Barberry, Elecampane, Garlic, Golden Seal, Green Tea, Myrrh, Oregano, Pau d'Arco, Pelargonium, Propolis, Rhubarb Root, Thyme

ANTICARIOGENIC

Green Tea, Licorice

ANTICATARRHAL

Elder Flower, Eyebright, Golden Rod, Golden Seal, Ground Ivy, Horseradish, Mullein, Ribwort

ANTICOAGULANT

Dan Shen

ANTICONVULSANT

Bacopa (mild), Kava, Paeonia

ANTIDEPRESSANT

Lavender, Schisandra (mild), St John's Wort

ANTIDIABETIC

See also Hypoglycaemic

Cinnamon, Goat's Rue, Gymnema

ANTIDIARRHOEAL

Cranesbill Root, Raspberry Leaf, Shatavari

ANTIECCHYMOTIC

Arnica (topically)

ANTIEMETIC

Barberry, Fringe Tree, Ginger, Globe Artichoke, Peppermint

ANTIFIBROTIC

Dan Shen, Gotu Kola

ANTIFUNGAL

Calendula (topically), Garlic, Oregano, Pau d'Arco, Pelargonium, Propolis, Stemona, Thuja, Thyme

ANTIHAEMORRHAGIC

Beth Root, Cranesbill Root, Golden Seal, Horsetail, Ladies Mantle, Rehmannia, Shepherd's Purse, Tienchi Ginseng, Yarrow

ANTIHYPERHIDROTIC

Sage

ANTI-INFLAMMATORY TOPICALLY

Arnica, Calendula, Chamomile, Comfrey, Evening Primrose Oil, Licorice, Myrrh, Oregon Grape, Witch Hazel Leaf, Yarrow

ANTI-INFLAMMATORY GASTROINTESTINAL

Baical Skullcap, Bilberry, Calendula, Chamomile, Fenugreek, Licorice, Meadowsweet, Yarrow

ANTI-INFLAMMATORY MUSCULOSKELETAL

See also Antirheumatic

Boswellia, Cat's Claw, Celery Seed, Devil's Claw, Ginger, Juniper, Polygonum cuspidatum, Rosehips, Turmeric, Willow Bark, Withania

ANTI-INFLAMMATORY AGAINST IMMUNE MEDIATED INFLAMMATION

See also Antiallergic, Immune depressant

Baical Skullcap, Bupleurum, Echinacea Root, Feverfew, Gotu Kola, Rehmannia, Sarsaparilla, Tylophora

ANTI-INFLAMMATORY, OTHER

Bearberry, Butcher's Broom, Crataeva, Dong Quai, Eyebright, Golden Rod, Golden Seal, Greater Celandine, Horsechestnut, Ladies Mantle, Paeonia, Poke Root, Rhubarb Root, Saw Palmetto, Tienchi Ginseng, Wild Yam

ANTILITHIC

Corn Silk, Crataeva, Gravel Root, Hydrangea

ANTIMICROBIAL

See also Antibacterial, Antifungal, Antiparasitic, Antiseptic, Antiviral

Aniseed, Barberry, Calendula, Cloves, Fennel, Golden Seal, Myrrh, Oregon Grape, Peppermint (internally and topically), Rosemary, Sage, St John's Wort, Thuja, Thyme, Yarrow

ANTIOBESITY

Bladderwrack, Coleus, Gymnema

ANTIOEDEMATOUS

Bilberry, Butcher's Broom, Horsechestnut

ANTIOXIDANT

Bacopa, Bilberry, Cat's Claw, Chaparral, Elder Berry, Garlic, Ginkgo, Grape Seed, Green Tea, Hawthorn (leaf & berry), Olive Leaf, Oregano, Polygonum cuspidatum, Polygonum multiflorum, Rhodiola, Rosemary, Sage, Schisandra, Thyme, St Mary's Thistle, Turmeric

ANTI-PAF

Ginkgo

ANTIPARASITIC

Barberry, Euphorbia, Garlic, Pau d'Arco, Propolis, Qing Hao, Wormwood

ANTIPLATELET

Coleus, Dan Shen, Dong Quai, Garlic, Ginger, Turmeric

ANTIPROSTATIC

Hydrangea, Nettle Root, Saw Palmetto, Willow Herb

ANTIPROTOZOAL

See Antiparasitic

ANTIPRURITIC

Kava (topically), Peppermint (topically)

ANTIPYRETIC

Baptisia, Qing Hao, Rehmannia, Rhubarb Root, Willow Bark, Yarrow

ANTIRHEUMATIC

Black Cohosh, Celery Seed, Chamomile, Dandelion Root, Devil's Claw, Nettle Leaf, Prickly Ash, Sarsaparilla, Wild Yam, Willow Bark

ANTISEPTIC

See Antibacterial, Antimicrobial, Urinary Antiseptic

ANTISPASMODIC

See Spasmolytic

ANTITHYROID

Bugleweed, Motherwort

ANTITUMOUR

Boswellia, Chaparral, Pau d'Arco, Polygonum cuspidatum, Red Clover (traditional use), Rhodiola, Sheep Sorrel, Shiitake, Violet Leaf (reputed)

ANTITUSSIVE

Bupleurum, Licorice, Peppermint, Schisandra, Stemona, Wild Cherry

ANTIULCER (PEPTIC)

Chamomile, Chickweed

ANTIURAEMIC

Rhubarb Root

ANTIVIRAL

Calendula (topically), Elder Berry, Greater Celandine (topically), Green Tea (topically), Lemon Balm (topically), Lomatium, Phyllanthus, Propolis, St John's Wort, Thuja

ANXIOLYTIC

Bacopa, California Poppy, Green Oats, Kava, Lavender, Mexican Valerian, Passionflower, Valerian, Zizyphus

APHRODISIAC

Shatavari, Tribulus Leaf

AROMATIC DIGESTIVE

Angelica Root, Chen Pi, Cinnamon, Cloves, Coleus, Dill, Ginger

ASTRINGENT

See also Antidiarrhoeal and Vulnerary

Agrimony (mild), Bayberry, Bearberry, Beth Root, Black Haw, Chickweed, Cinnamon, Cramp Bark, Cranberry, Cranesbill Root, Eyebright, Grape Seed, Green Tea, Ground Ivy, Hawthorn (leaf & berry) (mild), Horsetail, Ladies Mantle, Meadowsweet, Myrrh, Propolis, Raspberry Leaf, Ribwort, Rosehips, Sage, Squaw Vine, Vervain, Wild Cherry, Witch Hazel Leaf

BITTER TONIC

Also known as a Bitter

Barberry, Dandelion Root, Devil's Claw, Gentian, Globe Artichoke, Golden Seal, Hops, Olive Leaf, Polygonum multiflorum, Qing Hao, True Unicorn, White Horehound, Wood Betony, Wormwood, Yarrow

BLADDER TONIC

Crataeva

BRONCHOSPASMOLYTIC

Adhatoda, Black Haw, Coleus, Elecampane, Grindelia, Inula racemosa

CANCER PREVENTATIVE

See also Antitumour

Korean Ginseng

CARDIOPROTECTIVE

Dan Shen, Hawthorn (leaf & berry), Terminalia arjuna, Tienchi Ginseng

CARDIOTONIC

Astragalus, Coleus, Hawthorn (leaf & berry) (mild), Korean Ginseng, Motherwort

CARMINATIVE

Angelica Root, Aniseed, Cayenne, Chamomile, Chen Pi, Cinnamon, Cloves, Dill, Fennel, Ginger, Hyssop, Juniper, Lavender, Lemon Balm, Peppermint, Rosemary

CHOLAGOGUE

Barberry, Blue Flag, Butternut, Cloves, Dandelion Root, Fringe Tree, Gentian, Globe Artichoke, Greater Celandine, Peppermint, Yellow Dock

CHOLERETIC

Andrographis, Barberry, Bayberry (mild), Dandelion Leaf, Dandelion Root, Fringe Tree, Globe Artichoke, Golden Seal, Greater Celandine, Mugwort, St Mary's Thistle, Turmeric

CIRCULATORY STIMULANT

Bayberry, Cayenne, Ginger (peripheral), Ginkgo, Horseradish, Prickly Ash, Rosemary

CNS STIMULANT

Kola Nut

COGNITION ENHANCING

Bacopa, Ginkgo, Korean Ginseng, Paeonia

COLLAGEN STABILISING

Grape Seed, Hawthorn (leaf & berry)

COUNTERIRRITANT

Cayenne, Horseradish

DEMULCENT

See also Urinary demulcent

Chickweed, Comfrey, Fenugreek, Licorice, Marshmallow (root & leaf), Mullein, Ribwort, Slippery Elm, Sundew, Violet Leaf

DEPURATIVE

Black Walnut, Blue Flag, Burdock, Butternut, Clivers, Echinacea Root, Fringe Tree, Globe Artichoke, Golden Seal, Hemidesmus, Nettle Leaf, Oregon Grape, Pau d'Arco, Poke Root, Red Clover, Sarsaparilla, Thuja, Yellow Dock

DIAPHORETIC

Angelica Root, Bayberry, Boneset, Bupleurum, Cayenne, Chamomile, Chaparral, Elder Flower, Elecampane, Ginger, Golden Rod, Hemidesmus, Hyssop, Lemon Balm, Lime Flowers, Peppermint, Pleurisy Root, Prickly Ash, Vervain (mild), Violet Leaf, Yarrow

DIURETIC

Astragalus, Buchu (mild), Celery Seed, Corn Silk, Couch Grass (soothing), Dandelion Leaf, Dandelion Root, Globe Artichoke, Golden Rod, Gravel Root, Green Tea, Horsetail, Hydrangea, Juniper (mild), Kola Nut (mild), Shatavari, Terminalia arjuna (mild)

DIURETIC DEPURATIVE

Burdock, Celery Seed, Clivers, Globe Artichoke, Gravel Root

DOPAMINERGIC AGONIST

Chaste Tree

EMMENAGOGUE

Blue Cohosh, Feverfew (in high doses), Motherwort, Mugwort

EMOLLIENT

See also Demulcent

Marshmallow (root & leaf), Slippery Elm

EXPECTORANT

Adhatoda, Angelica Root, Aniseed, Beth Root (mild), Chen Pi, Elecampane, Fennel, Grindelia, Ground Ivy, Hyssop, Licorice, Mullein, Pelargonium, Pleurisy Root, Polygala, Sundew, Thyme, Violet Leaf, White Horehound

FEMALE TONIC

Dong Quai

GALACTAGOGUE

Aniseed, Chaste Tree, Fennel, Fenugreek, Goat's Rue, Shatavari, Vervain

HEALING PROMOTER

Gotu Kola

HEPATOPROTECTIVE

Andrographis, Bupleurum, Dan Shen, Globe Artichoke, Phyllanthus, St Mary's Thistle, Rosemary, Schisandra, Terminalia arjuna

HEPATOTROPHORESTORATIVE

Globe Artichoke, St Mary's Thistle

HYPNOTIC

California Poppy, Corydalis, Hops, Kava, Mexican Valerian, Passionflower, Valerian, Zizyphus

HYPOCHOLESTEROLAEMIC

See also Hypolipidaemic

Albizia, Fenugreek, Garlic, Globe Artichoke, Green Tea, Gymnema, Polygonum multiflorum, Terminalia arjuna, Tienchi Ginseng

HYPOGLYCAEMIC

Fenugreek, Goat's Rue, Gymnema, Phyllanthus

HYPOLIPIDAEMIC

See also Hypocholesterolaemic

Fenugreek, Globe Artichoke, Gymnema, Turmeric

HYPOTENSIVE

See also Peripheral vasodilator

Astragalus, Black Haw, Coleus, Cramp Bark, Dan Shen, Evening Primrose Oil, Garlic, Hawthorn (leaf & berry), Inula racemosa, Mistletoe, Motherwort, Olive Leaf, Zizyphus

IMMUNE DEPRESSANT

Hemidesmus, Tylophora

IMMUNE ENHANCING

Andrographis, Astragalus, Baptisia, Cat's Claw, Echinacea Root, Elder Berry, Pau d'Arco, Poke Root

IMMUNE MODULATING

Echinacea Root, Korean Ginseng, Pelargonium, Reishi, Sheep Sorrel, Shiitake, Siberian Ginseng, Withania

LAXATIVE

Aloes Resin, Blue Flag, Butternut, Cascara, Damiana (mild), Dandelion Leaf, Dandelion Root, Dong Quai (mild), Fringe Tree (mild), Greater Celandine (mild), Licorice (mild), Rhubarb Root, Senna Pods, Slippery Elm, Yellow Dock (mild)

LOCAL ANAESTHETIC

Kava

LYMPHATIC

Baptisia, Blue Flag, Calendula, Clivers, Echinacea Root, Myrrh, Poke Root

MALE TONIC

Korean Ginseng, Saw Palmetto

METABOLIC STIMULANT

Cayenne, Horseradish

MUCOPROTECTIVE

Licorice, Meadowsweet

MUCOUS MEMBRANE TONIC

Eyebright

MUCOUS MEMBRANE TROPHORESTORATIVE

Golden Seal

NERVINE TONIC

Bacopa, Damiana, Gotu Kola, Green Oats, Motherwort, Oats Seed, Pasque Flower, Polygonum multiflorum, Schisandra, Skullcap, St John's Wort, Vervain

NEUROPROTECTIVE

Ginkgo

NUTRIENT

Alfalfa, Evening Primrose Oil

OESTROGEN MODULATING

Alfalfa, Aniseed, Black Cohosh, Fennel, False Unicorn Root, Hops, Paeonia, Wild Yam

OREXIGENIC

Fennel, Fenugreek, Mugwort

OVARIAN TONIC

Blue Cohosh, False Unicorn Root

OXYTOCIC

Adhatoda, Blue Cohosh, Golden Seal (reputed), Schisandra

PARTURIFACIENT

See also Oxytocic

Raspberry Leaf, Squaw Vine

PARTUS PREPARATOR

Raspberry Leaf, Squaw Vine

PERIPHERAL VASODILATOR

Cramp Bark, Hawthorn (leaf & berry), Lime Flowers, Mistletoe, Yarrow

PROGESTEROGENIC

Chaste Tree (indirectly)

PROLACTIN INHIBITOR

Chaste Tree

PUNGENT

Cayenne, Ginger, Horseradish

REFRIGERANT

Chickweed

RUBEFACIENT

See also Counterirritant

Thyme

SEDATIVE (MILD)

Bugleweed, California Poppy, Chamomile, Cramp Bark, Corydalis, Hops, Hyssop, Jamaica Dogwood, Kava, Lemon Balm, Lime Flowers, Mexican Valerian, Mistletoe, Passionflower, Peppermint, Polygala, Skullcap, True Unicorn, Valerian, Wild Cherry, Withania, Wood Betony, Zizyphus

SEXUAL TONIC

Shatavari

SIALAGOGUE

Echinacea Root, Gentian, Prickly Ash

SKELETAL MUSCLE RELAXANT

Kava, Paeonia (mild)

SPASMOLYTIC

Aniseed, Black Cohosh, Blue Cohosh, Cayenne, Chamomile, Cinnamon, Cloves, Coleus, Corydalis, Cramp Bark, Elecampane, Fennel, Greater Celandine, Hops, Hyssop, Inula racemosa, Jamaica Dogwood, Kava, Lavender, Lemon Balm, Lime Flowers, Mexican Valerian, Motherwort, Paeonia, Pasque Flower, Passionflower, Peppermint, Rosemary, Sage, Saw Palmetto, Shatavari, Skullcap, Squaw Vine, Sundew, Thyme, True Unicorn, Valerian, White Horehound, Wild Yam, Yarrow

STYPTIC (HAEMOSTATIC)

See also Vulnerary

Calendula, Cranesbill, Horsetail, Nettle Leaf, Rhubarb Root, Ribwort, Shepherd's Purse, Witch Hazel Leaf, Yarrow

THYMOLEPTIC

Kola Nut, Oats Seed, Vervain

THYROID STIMULANT

Bacopa, Bladderwrack

TISSUE PERFUSION ENHANCING

Ginkgo

TONIC

Also known as general body tonic

See also other specific body tonics

Astragalus, Codonopsis, Damiana, Korean Ginseng, Oats Seed, Reishi, Rhodiola, Shatavari, Tribulus Leaf, Withania

TSH ANTAGONIST

Lemon Balm

URINARY ANTISEPTIC

Bearberry, Buchu, Juniper, Meadowsweet (mild), Shepherd's Purse

URINARY DEMULCENT

Corn Silk, Couch Grass

UTERINE ANTIHAEMORRHAGIC

See also Antihaemorrhagic

Beth Root, Ladies Mantle, Shepherd's Purse, Tienchi ginseng

UTERINE SPASMOLYTIC

Black Cohosh, Black Haw, Blue Cohosh, Cramp Bark, Motherwort, Paeonia, Pasque Flower, Wild Yam

UTERINE TONIC

Beth Root, Black Cohosh, Blue Cohosh, False Unicorn Root, True Unicorn

VASOPROTECTIVE

Bilberry, Grape Seed

VENOTONIC

Butcher's Broom, Grape Seed, Horsechestnut

VULNERARY

See also Antiulcer, Astringent, Demulcent

Calendula, Chamomile, Comfrey, Cranesbill, Dan Shen, Echinacea Root, Golden Seal, Gotu Kola, Greater Celandine (topically), Mullein, Myrrh, Propolis, Ribwort, St John's Wort, Yarrow

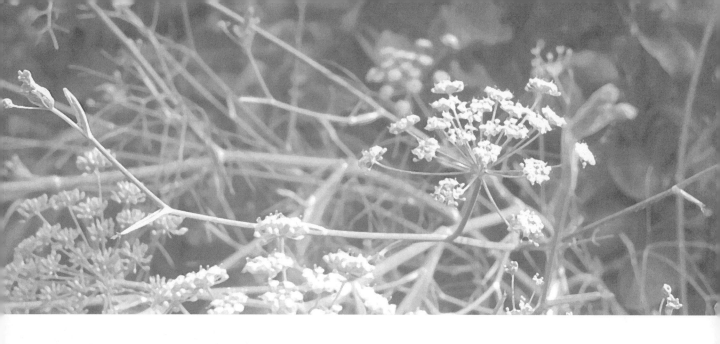

Therapeutic Index

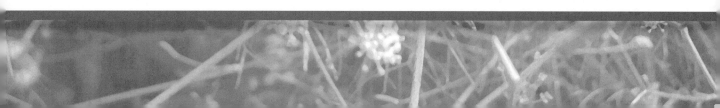

ABDOMINAL BLOATING

See also Colic

Key   Chen Pi, Cloves, Gentian, Ginger, Globe Artichoke, St Mary's Thistle, Wormwood

ACHLORHYDRIA

See Hypochlorhydria

ACNE

Key   Andrographis, Blue Flag, Burdock, Calendula, Chaste Tree (male and female), Clivers, Golden Seal, Licorice (topically), Oregon Grape

Other   Dan Shen, Nettle Leaf

ACNE, TOPICALLY

Key   Calendula, Oregon Grape, Poke Root

Other   Barberry, Golden Seal

ADDISON'S DISEASE

See also Autoimmune disease

Key   Licorice

ADENOMYOSIS

See also Endometriosis and Dysmenorrhoea

Key   Dong Quai, False Unicorn, Ladies Mantle, Paeonia

Other   Chaste Tree

ADHD

Key   Bacopa, Ginkgo, Korean Ginseng, Paeonia, Rhodiola, Withania

Other   Grape Seed, Rosemary, Schisandra, Siberian Ginseng, Skullcap, St John's Wort

ADHESIONS, TO PREVENT

Key   Gotu Kola

ADRENAL DEPLETION

Key   Licorice, Rehmannia

Other   Rhodiola, Siberian Ginseng, Skullcap, St John's Wort, Withania

AGEING, TO SLOW THE PROCESS

See also Alzheimer's disease

Key   Echinacea Root (immunological), Garlic, Green Tea, Korean Ginseng, Polygonum cuspidatum, Polygonum multiflorum, Reishi

Other   Bilberry, Rosemary

AIDS/HIV

Key   Astragalus, Cat's Claw

Other   Korean Ginseng (adjunct therapy), Reishi, Rhodiola (adjunct therapy), Sheep Sorrel, Shiitake, Withania (adjunct therapy)

ALLERGIC RHINITIS

See Hay fever

ALTITUDE SICKNESS

Key   Ginkgo (controversial)

ALZHEIMER'S DISEASE

Key   Bacopa, Ginkgo

Other   Grape Seed, Ginger, Korean Ginseng, Paeonia, Rosemary, Sage, Turmeric

ALZHEIMER'S DISEASE, TO PREVENT

Key   Ginkgo, Green Tea, Turmeric

Other   Bilberry, Grape Seed, Rosemary

AMALGAM POISONING

See Heavy metal burden

AMENORRHOEA, PRIMARY

Key   Chaste Tree, Tribulus

AMENORRHOEA, SECONDARY

See also Polycystic Ovary Syndrome

Key   Chaste Tree, Dong Quai, False Unicorn, Fennel, Motherwort

Other   Blue Cohosh, Mugwort

ANAEMIA, DEFICIENT BLOOD

Key   Codonopsis, Dong Quai, Withania

ANAEMIA, DEFICIENT IRON

Key   Withania

ANAESTHESIA, TO REDUCE TOXIC EFFECTS

Key   St Mary's Thistle

ANAL FISSURE, TO SOFTEN STOOL

Key   Aloes Resin, Cascara, Senna Pods, Slippery Elm

ANDROGEN EXCESS

Key   Chaste Tree (male, high doses), Licorice (female), Paeonia (female)

Other   Hops (male)

ANGINA PECTORIS

Key — Coleus, Dan Shen, Dong Quai, Ginger, Hawthorn, Inula racemosa, Lime Flowers, Mistletoe, Olive Leaf, Terminalia arjuna, Tienchi Ginseng, Turmeric

Other — Astragalus, Cayenne, Paeonia

ANKYLOSING SPONDYLITIS

See also Autoimmune Disease and Bowel flora

Key — Boswellia, Celery Seed, Willow Bark

ANOREXIA

Key — Angelica Root, Chen Pi, Cinnamon, Codonopsis, Dandelion Root, Devil's Claw, Fennel, Fenugreek, Gentian, Globe Artichoke, Hops, Mugwort, True Unicorn, Vervain, White Horehound, Wormwood, Yarrow

ANXIETY

Key — Bacopa, California Poppy, Corydalis, Damiana, Hawthorn (mild), Hops, Jamaica Dogwood, Kava, Lavender, Lemon Balm, Lime Flowers, Mexican Valerian, Oats Green, Passionflower, Skullcap, St John's Wort, Valerian, Vervain, Wood Betony, Zizyphus (especially with excessive sweating)

Other — Chamomile, Gotu Kola, Motherwort

APPETITE, POOR

See Anorexia

ARRHYTHMIAS, CARDIAC

Key — Corydalis, Hawthorn, Motherwort, Terminalia arjuna, Tienchi Ginseng

Other — Dong Quai

ASTHMA

Key — Adhatoda, Albizia, Baical Skullcap, Boswellia, Coleus, Elecampane, Euphorbia, Ginger, Ginkgo (anti PAF), Grindelia, Hyssop, Inula racemosa, Licorice, Marshmallow Root, Polygala, Rehmannia, Sundew, Turmeric, Tylophora, Violet Leaf, White Horehound

Other — Andrographis (immune support), Black Haw, Cat's Claw (immune support), Elder Flower (with sinusitis), Eyebright (with sinusitis), Feverfew, Passionflower

ATHEROSCLEROSIS, TO TREAT AND PREVENT

Key — Garlic, Ginkgo, Globe Artichoke, Grape Seed, Green Tea, Hawthorn, Polygonum cuspidatum, Turmeric

ATHLETE'S FOOT

See Tinea

AUTOIMMUNE DISEASE

Key — Astragalus, Bupleurum, Echinacea Root (controversial), Hemidesmus, Rehmannia, Tylophora, Wormwood

Other — Cat's Claw, Feverfew, Reishi, Shiitake, St John's Wort

BACK PAIN, LOWER BACK

See also Osteoarthritis and Disc prolapse

Key — Boswellia, Devil's Claw, Willow Bark

Other — Horsechestnut (for sciatica), St John's Wort (for sciatica)

BED SORES

See also Healing

Key — Calendula (topically), Echinacea Root (also topically)

BED WETTING

See Enuresis

BELL'S PALSY

Key — Ginkgo, Gotu Kola, Grape Seed, Horsechestnut, St John's Wort

BENIGN PROSTATIC HYPERPLASIA

Key — Crataeva (hypotonic bladder), Horsetail, Hydrangea, Nettle Root, Saw Palmetto, Willow Herb

Other — Corydalis, Cramp Bark

BILIOUSNESS

See Nausea

BLADDER INFECTION

See Cystitis

BLADDER STONES

Key — Bearberry, Crataeva, Golden Rod, Gravel Root, Hydrangea

BLADDER, ATONIC

Key — Crataeva

BLEEDING, INTERNAL

Key   Cranesbill Root, Horsetail, Rehmannia, Shepherd's Purse, Tienchi Ginseng, Yarrow

BLEEDING, SKIN

See Wounds, topically

BLEPHARITIS

See also Rosacea and Infection, chronic

Key   Eyebright, Fennel (topically), Golden Seal

BOILS

See Furunculosis

BOWEL FLORA, TO MODIFY

Key   Aniseed, Garlic, Golden Seal, Grape Seed, Green Tea, Oregano, Slippery Elm

Other   Barberry, Marshmallow Root

BREAST FEEDING

See Lactation

BREAST GROWTHS, BENIGN

Key   Chaste Tree, Echinacea Root, Paeonia, Thuja

Other   Blue Cohosh

BREAST TENDERNESS

See Mastalgia

BRONCHIAL ASTHMA

Key   Adhatoda, Aniseed, Echinacea Root, Elecampane, Euphorbia, Fennel, Garlic, Ginger, Grindelia, Hyssop, Inula racemosa, Licorice, Oregano, Thyme

Other   Pelargonium

BRONCHIECTASIS

Key   Astragalus, Echinacea Root, Elecampane, Ginger, Golden Seal, Mullein, Oregano, Polygala, Ribwort, Thyme

Other   Garlic, Pelargonium

BRONCHITIS, ACUTE

Key   Adhatoda (acute doses), Andrographis (acute doses), Aniseed, Echinacea Root (acute doses), Elder Flower, Elecampane, Ginger, Hyssop, Licorice, Marshmallow Root, Mullein, Pelargonium, Pleurisy Root, Polygala, Sundew, Thyme, White Horehound, Wild Cherry

Other   Angelica Root, Fennel

BRONCHITIS, CHRONIC

Key   Adhatoda, Aniseed, Coleus, Elecampane, Euphorbia, Fennel, Garlic, Ginger, Golden Seal, Grindelia, Ground Ivy, Hyssop, Inula racemosa (with cardiac complications), Licorice, Marshmallow Root, Mullein, Myrrh, Oregano, Pelargonium, Polygala, Ribwort, Sundew, Thyme, Violet Leaf, White Horehound, Wild Cherry

BRUISE EASILY

Key   Bilberry, Butcher's Broom, Gotu Kola, Grape Seed, Horsechestnut

BRUISES

Key   Arnica (topically), Butcher's Broom, Grape Seed, Horsechestnut (also topically)

BUERGER'S DISEASE

Key   Angelica Root, Dan Shen, Dong Quai, Echinacea Root, Garlic, Ginger, Ginkgo, Gotu Kola, Hawthorn, Prickly Ash

BURNS

Key   Calendula (topically), Chickweed (topically), Echinacea Root, Gotu Kola (also topically), Marshmallow Root (topically), Propolis (topically)

CACHEXIA

See also Anorexia

Key   Codonopsis, Gentian, Korean Ginseng, Rhodiola, Siberian Ginseng, St Mary's Thistle, Tribulus, Withania, Wormwood

CALCULI

See Kidney Stones

CANCER, ADJUNCT THERAPY

See also during chemotherapy and radiotherapy

Key Cat's Claw, Chaparral, Green Tea (preventative also), Korean Ginseng (preventative also), Pau D'Arco, Reishi, Sheep Sorrel, Shiitake, Willow Herb (prostate)

Other Boswellia, Codonopsis, Poke Root (especially breast and uterus), Propolis, Red Clover Flower, Thuja (controversial), Turmeric (preventative also), Violet Leaf

CANCER, DURING CHEMOTHERAPY

Key Astragalus, Korean Ginseng, Reishi, Rhodiola, Sheep Sorrel, Shiitake, Siberian Ginseng, Withania

Other Baical Skullcap, Dan Shen (for lymphoma), Echinacea Root, St Mary's Thistle

CANCER, DURING RADIOTHERAPY

Key Astragalus, Grape Seed (following radiotherapy, not during), Korean Ginseng, Reishi, Rhodiola, Sheep Sorrel, Shiitake, Siberian Ginseng, Withania

Other Echinacea Root

CANDIDIASIS, GASTROINTESTINAL

See also Infection, gastrointestinal

Key Andrographis, Aniseed, Barberry, Echinacea Root, Garlic, Golden Seal, Grape Seed, Green Tea, Oregano, Pau D'Arco, St Mary's Thistle

CANDIDIASIS, VAGINAL

See also Infection, chronic

Key Andrographis, Chaste Tree, Echinacea Root, Pau D'Arco (also topically)

Other Aniseed (topically), Oregano (topically), Thyme (topically)

CANKER SORES

See Ulcers, mouth

CAPILLARY FRAGILITY

Key Bilberry, Ginkgo, Grape Seed

Other Butcher's Broom, Gotu Kola, Horsechestnut

CARDIAC FAILURE, MILD CONGESTIVE

Key Astragalus, Coleus, Hawthorn, Korean Ginseng, Terminalia arjuna

CARDIOMYOPATHY

Key Dan Shen, Hawthorn, Terminalia arjuna

CARDIOVASCULAR DISEASE PREVENTION OF

Key Garlic, Green Tea, Polygonum cuspidatum, Rosemary

Other Coleus, Grape Seed, Turmeric

CARPAL TUNNEL SYNDROME

Key Butcher's Broom, Grape Seed, Horsechestnut, St John's Wort

CATARACT, TO PREVENT DETERIORATION

Key Bilberry, Grape Seed, Ginkgo, Turmeric

CATARRH, LOWER RESPIRATORY

Key Echinacea Root, Elecampane, Euphorbia, Garlic, Golden Seal, Grindelia, Mullein, Ribwort

CATARRH, SINUS OR NASOPHARYNGEAL

Key Echinacea Root, Elder Flower, Eyebright, Fennel, Golden Rod, Golden Seal, Grindelia, Ground Ivy, Horseradish, Hyssop, Myrrh, Peppermint, Poke Root (chronic), Ribwort, Thyme, Violet Leaf (chronic)

Other Boneset

CATARRHAL DEAFNESS

Key Elder Flower, Eyebright, Golden Rod, Golden Seal, Ground Ivy, Ribwort

CELLULITIS

Key Andrographis (acute doses), Echinacea Root (acute doses), Gotu Kola (also topically), Grape Seed

CEREBROVASCULAR DISEASE

Key Dan Shen, Dong Quai, Ginkgo, Prickly Ash, Rosemary

Other Bacopa

CHEMOTHERAPY

See Cancer, during chemotherapy

CHILBLAINS

Key   Calendula (topically), Cayenne, Ginger, Ginkgo, Prickly Ash

CHLOASMA

Key   Grape Seed

CHOLECYSTITIS

Key   Andrographis (acute doses), Barberry, Dandelion Leaf, Dandelion Root, Echinacea Root (acute doses), Fringe Tree, Globe Artichoke, Greater Celandine

CHOLELITHIASIS

See Gall stones

CHRONIC FATIGUE SYNDROME

Key   Astragalus, Ginkgo, Hawthorn, Korean Ginseng, Licorice, Lomatium, Rehmannia, Rhodiola, St John's Wort, Withania

Other   Boswellia, Cat's Claw, Codonopsis, Echinacea Root, Evening Primrose Oil, Reishi, Schisandra, Shiitake, Siberian Ginseng

CHRONIC LYMPHOCYTIC LEUKAEMIA

Key   Green Tea, Echinacea Root

CHRONIC STRESS

See Stress

CIRCULATION, PERIPHERAL IMPAIRED

Key   Cayenne, Dan Shen, Dong Quai, Garlic, Ginger, Ginkgo, Grape Seed, Hawthorn, Prickly Ash

COGNITIVE PERFORMANCE, TO IMPROVE

Key   Bacopa, Ginkgo, Korean Ginseng, Paeonia, Rhodiola, Rosemary, Sage, Schisandra, Siberian Ginseng

Other   Gotu Kola

COLD SORES

See Herpes simplex

COLDS

See Common cold

COLIC, FLATULENT

See also Bowel flora and Flatulence

Key   Aniseed, Cayenne, Chamomile, Chen Pi, Cinnamon, Cloves, Dandelion Root, Dill, Fennel, Gentian, Ginger, Globe Artichoke, Lavender, Lemon Balm, Peppermint, St Mary's Thistle, Wormwood

COLIC, INFANTILE

Key   Aniseed, Chamomile, Dill, Fennel, Lemon Balm, Peppermint, Vervain

COLIC, INTESTINAL

Key   Aniseed, Chamomile, Chen Pi, Cramp Bark, Corydalis, Dill, Fennel, Gentian, Ginger, Lavender, Lemon Balm, Peppermint, Valerian, Wild Yam, Wormwood, Yarrow

COLIC, RENAL

See Kidney stones

COLITIS

See Ulcerative colitis

COMMON COLD

See also Infection, acute

Key   Andrographis (acute doses), Bayberry, Echinacea Root (acute doses), Elder Berry (acute doses), Elder Flower, Elecampane, Eyebright, Garlic, Ginger, Horseradish, Hyssop, Lime Flowers (acute doses), Lomatium, Mullein, Myrrh, Pelargonium, Peppermint, Pleurisy Root, Propolis, Thuja, Thyme, Violet Leaf, White Horehound (acute doses), Wild Cherry, Yarrow (acute doses)

Other   Bupleurum, Cinnamon, Lemon Balm, Meadowsweet, Wormwood

CONCENTRATION, TO ENHANCE

Key   Bacopa, Ginkgo, Korean Ginseng, Paeonia, Rhodiola, Rosemary, Sage, Schisandra, Siberian Ginseng

Other   Gotu Kola

CONJUNCTIVITIS

See also Infection or Hay Fever

Key Echinacea Root, Eyebright (also topically), Fennel (topically), Golden Seal, Raspberry Leaf (topically), Ribwort

CONNECTIVE TISSUE REPAIR

See Healing

CONNECTIVE TISSUE, TO STRENGTHEN

Key Grape Seed, Hawthorn, Polygonum multiflorum

CONSTIPATION

Key Aloes Resin, Butternut, Cascara, Damiana, Dandelion Leaf, Dandelion Root, Fringe Tree, Gentian, Globe Artichoke, Licorice, Marshmallow Root, Polygonum cuspidatum, Rehmannia, Rhubarb Root, Senna Pods, Slippery Elm, St Mary's Thistle, Yellow Dock

CONVALESCENCE

Key Cat's Claw, Codonopsis, Fenugreek, Gentian, Korean Ginseng, Licorice, Rehmannia, Reishi, Rhodiola, Siberian Ginseng, Tribulus Leaf, Withania

Other Fringe Tree, Golden Seal

CORONARY

See Heart attack

COUGH

Key Elecampane, Fennel, Grindelia, Ground Ivy, Licorice, Marshmallow Root, Mullein, Peppermint, Pleurisy Root, Ribwort, Stemona, Thyme, Violet Leaf, Wild Cherry

Other Aniseed (spasmodic), Bupleurum (chronic)

CRAMPS, LEG

Key Ginkgo, Horsechestnut, Kava, Prickly Ash

Other Butcher's Broom, Gotu Kola, Paeonia

CROHN'S DISEASE

See also Autoimmune disease and Bowel flora

Key Boswellia, Echinacea Root, Golden Seal, Slippery Elm, Wormwood

CYSTIC FIBROSIS

See also Catarrh, lower respiratory and Digestive weakness

Key Turmeric, Boswellia

CYSTIC HYPERPLASIA, OF THE ENDOMETRIUM

Key Chaste Tree, False Unicorn

CYSTITIS

Key Andrographis (acute doses), Bearberry, Buchu (acute doses), Corn Silk (acute doses), Couch Grass (acute doses), Cranberry (acute doses), Crataeva, Echinacea Root (acute doses), Golden Rod, Horsetail, Hydrangea, Juniper (acute doses), Marshmallow Root, Saw Palmetto, Shepherd's Purse (acute doses)

Other Licorice (acute doses), Meadowsweet

CYSTITIS, RECURRENT

Key Andrographis, Buchu, Bearberry, Cranberry, Crataeva, Echinacea Root, Juniper

Other Licorice

DEAFNESS, ACUTE

See Hearing loss, idiopathic

DEBILITY

Key Alfalfa, Astragalus, Cat's Claw, Codonopsis, Dong Quai (secondary to breast feeding), Fenugreek, Gentian, Kola Nut (short-term use), Korean Ginseng, Oats Seed, Polygonum multiflorum (in the elderly), Rhodiola, Rosemary, Sarsaparilla, Schisandra, Shatavari (sexual), Siberian Ginseng, Withania

Other Fringe Tree

DEEP VEIN THROMBOSIS (DVT), TO REDUCE RISK

Key   Butcher's Broom, Coleus, Dan Shen, Dong Quai, Garlic, Ginger, Gotu Kola, Horsechestnut, Turmeric

DEMENTIA

See Alzheimer's disease

DEMENTIA, VASCULAR

See also Alzheimer's disease

Key   Bacopa, Ginkgo (prevention and treatment)

DENTAL CARIES, TO PREVENT

Key   Cloves (topically), Echinacea Root (also topically), Green Tea (topically)

DEPRESSION

Key   Damiana, Lavender (mild), Lemon Balm, Oats Green (mild), Oats Seed (mild), Siberian Ginseng (mild), St John's Wort, Vervain (mild)

Other   Kola Nut (with general muscular weakness), Skullcap, Valerian

DEPRESSION, POST NATAL

See also Depression

Key   Chaste Tree

DERMATITIS (ECZEMA)

Key   Albizia, Baical Skullcap, Blue Flag, Burdock, Butternut, Clivers, Echinacea Root, Evening Primrose Oil, Nettle Leaf, Oregon Grape, Poke Root, Red Clover Flower, Sarsaparilla, Yellow Dock

Other   Feverfew

DERMATITIS (ECZEMA), TOPICALLY

Key   Agrimony, Calendula, Chamomile, Chickweed, Comfrey, Golden Seal, Gotu Kola, Licorice, Oats Seed (as a decoction), Witch Hazel Leaf, Yarrow

DIABETES, MELLITUS

Key   Cinnamon, Fenugreek, Goat's Rue, Gymnema, Korean Ginseng (type 2), Phyllanthus (type 2), St Mary's Thistle (type 2)

DIABETES, GESTATIONAL

See also Diabetes mellitus

Key   Gymnema, St Mary's Thistle

DIABETIC NEUROPATHY

See also Diabetes mellitus

Key   Cayenne (topically), Evening Primrose Oil, Gotu Kola

Other   Baical Skullcap (to prevent), Dan Shen

DIABETIC RETINOPATHY

See also Diabetes mellitus

Key   Bilberry, Grape Seed

DIAPER RASH

See Nappy Rash

DIARRHOEA

Key   Agrimony (mild), Bayberry, Chamomile, Chen Pi, Cinnamon, Cranesbill, Fennel, Green Tea, Grape Seed, Meadowsweet, Raspberry Leaf, Rosehips, Thyme, Witch Hazel Leaf

Other   Ladies Mantle, Mullein

DIGESTIVE WEAKNESS

Key   Angelica Root, Cayenne, Chen Pi, Cinnamon, Coleus, Gentian, Ginger, Mugwort, Wormwood

DISC PROLAPSE/LESIONS

Key   Bilberry, California Poppy (acute doses for pain), Ginkgo, Gotu Kola, Grape Seed, Horsechestnut, Jamaica Dogwood (for pain), St John's Wort (for sciatica)

DIVERTICULITIS/DIVERTICULOSIS

See also Bowel flora

Key   Echinacea Root, Garlic, Golden Seal, Marshmallow Root, Slippery Elm, Wild Yam

DIZZINESS

See also Hypotension, postural

Key   Ginkgo, Wood Betony

Other   Polygonum multiflorum

DRUG ABUSE/ADDICTION

Key   California Poppy, Kava, Korean Ginseng, Oats Green (controversial), Oats Seed (controversial), Passionflower, Siberian Ginseng, Skullcap, St John's Wort, Valerian, Withania

DUODENAL ULCER

See Ulcer, peptic

DYSBIOSIS

See Bowel flora

DYSENTERY

See also Infection, gastrointestinal

Key   Andrographis (acute doses), Echinacea Root (acute doses), Euphorbia (amoebic, acute doses), Rhubarb Root

DYSGLYCAEMIA

Key   Ginkgo, Gymnema (lower doses), Licorice, Rehmannia, Schisandra, Siberian Ginseng, Withania

DYSMENORRHOEA, CONGESTIVE

Key   Butcher's Broom, Chaste Tree, Corydalis, Dong Quai, Ginkgo, Grape Seed, Horsechestnut

DYSMENORRHOEA, SPASMODIC

Key   Black Cohosh, Black Haw (acute doses), Blue Cohosh, Calendula, Corydalis (acute doses), Cramp Bark (acute doses), Dong Quai, False Unicorn, Fennel, Ginger (acute doses), Jamaica Dogwood, Motherwort, Paeonia, Pasque Flower, Raspberry Leaf (acute doses), Squaw Vine, Wild Yam

Other   Bilberry, Mugwort, Passionflower, Valerian

DYSPEPSIA

See also Nervous dyspepsia

Key   Angelica Root, Aniseed, Barberry, Chen Pi, Cinnamon, Cloves, Dandelion Leaf, Dandelion Root, Devil's Claw (20 mL per week/1:2), Fennel, Fenugreek, Fringe Tree, Ginger, Globe Artichoke, Greater Celandine, Meadowsweet, Peppermint, Sage, St Mary's Thistle, Thyme, True Unicorn, Turmeric, White Horehound, Yarrow

DYSURIA

See also Cystitis

Key   Bearberry (acute doses), Buchu (acute doses), Corn Silk (acute doses), Couch Grass (acute doses), Gravel Root, Horsetail, Hydrangea, Juniper (acute doses), Marshmallow Root

Other   Clivers, Meadowsweet

EARACHE

See also Catarrh, nasopharyngeal

Key   Mullein (infused oil)

ECZEMA

See Dermatitis

EDEMA

See Oedema

ELDERLY, TONIC FOR

Key   Bacopa, Ginkgo, Korean Ginseng, Polygonum multiflorum, Reishi, Rhodiola, Siberian Ginseng, Tribulus, Withania

EMACIATION

See also Cachexia

Key   Codonopsis, Korean Ginseng, Rhodiola, Siberian Ginseng, Tribulus, Withania

EMPHYSEMA

See also Bronchitis, chronic

Key   Coleus, Elecampane, Euphorbia, Gotu Kola, Grape Seed, Green Tea, Horsetail

ENDOMETRIOSIS

See also Dysmenorrhoea

Key   Calendula, Chaste Tree (higher doses), Cramp Bark, Dong Quai, Ginger, Ladies Mantle, Paeonia

Other   Blue Cohosh, Bupleurum, Gotu Kola, Pasque Flower, Rehmannia, Rhubarb Root

THERAPEUTICS

ENURESIS NOCTURIA

Key   Corn Silk, Crataeva, Horsetail, Schisandra, St John's Wort, Thyme

EPILEPSY

Key   Bacopa, Hyssop (petit mal), Kava, Mexican Valerian, Mistletoe, Paeonia, Passionflower, Skullcap, Valerian

EPISTAXIS

Key   Rehmannia, Shepherd's Purse (topically), Yarrow

Other   Grape Seed, Horsetail, Nettle Leaf

ESTROGEN, LOW

See Oestrogen, low

ESTROGEN, RELATIVE EXCESS

See Oestrogen, relative excess

EXCITABILITY

Key   Hops, Kava, Lavender, Mexican Valerian, Mistletoe, Pasque Flower, Passionflower, Polygala, Skullcap, Valerian

EXERCISE, TO HELP PERFORMANCE

Key   Korean Ginseng, Rhodiola, Schisandra, Siberian Ginseng, Tribulus Leaf, Withania

EXHAUSTION

See Fatigue

EYE STRAIN

Key   Bilberry

EYES, DRY

Key   Eyebright, Golden Seal, Ribwort

FAILURE TO THRIVE

See also Cachexia

Key   Gentian, Korean Ginseng, Rhodiola, Withania

FATIGUE

Key   Astragalus, Codonopsis, Kola Nut, Korean Ginseng, Licorice, Oats Green (especially nervous), Oats Seed (especially nervous), Polygonum multiflorum (with insomnia), Rehmannia, Rhodiola, Sage, Sarsaparilla, Schisandra, Siberian Ginseng, Skullcap (nervous), St John's Wort, Tribulus Leaf, Withania

FERTILITY FEMALE, TO ENHANCE

See also Polycystic ovary syndrome

Key   Black Cohosh, Chaste Tree, Cramp Bark, Dong Quai, False Unicorn, Licorice, Paeonia, Saw Palmetto, Shatavari, Siberian Ginseng, Tribulus Leaf, True Unicorn (controversial), Wild Yam

FERTILITY MALE, TO ENHANCE

Key   Korean Ginseng, Saw Palmetto, Shatavari, Tribulus Leaf, Withania

FEVER

Key   Cayenne, Ginger, Hyssop, Lime Flowers, Pleurisy Root, Rehmannia, Vervain, Willow Bark, Yarrow (generally all acute doses)

Other   Lemon Balm, Meadowsweet, Sage

FIBROCYSTIC BREAST DISEASE

See Breast growths, benign

FIBROIDS, UTERINE

See also Menorrhagia

Key   Chaste Tree, Echinacea Root, Ladies Mantle, Paeonia, Rosemary, Schisandra, Thuja

FIBROMYALGIA

Key   Astragalus, Bupleurum, Celery Seed, Ginkgo, Hawthorn, Korean Ginseng, Rehmannia, Rhodiola, St John's Wort, Withania

Other   Boswellia, Cat's Claw, Chaste Tree, Codonopsis, Echinacea Root, Reishi, Shiitake, Siberian Ginseng, Willow Bark

FLATULENCE

See also Bowel flora

Key   Andrographis, Angelica Root, Aniseed, Chamomile, Cloves, Dill, Fennel, Gentian, Globe Artichoke, Lemon Balm, Peppermint, Sage, St Mary's Thistle, White Horehound, Wormwood

FOOD ALLERGIES/SENSITIVITIES

See also Digestive Weakness and Liver insufficiency (both types)

Key   Albizia, Andrographis, Baical Skullcap, Chamomile, Chen Pi, Echinacea Root, Gentian, Ginger, Globe Artichoke, St Mary's Thistle, Wormwood

FRACTURES, TO PROMOTE HEALING

Key   Comfrey (topically), Dan Shen, Gotu Kola

FUNGAL INFECTION

See Tinea or Candidiasis

FURUNCULOSIS

Key   Andrographis, Burdock, Echinacea Root, Marshmallow Root (topically), Poke Root

Other   Arnica (topically), Baptisia

GALL BLADDER DYSFUNCTION

Key   Barberry, Dandelion Root, Fringe Tree, Globe Artichoke, Greater Celandine, Peppermint

GALL BLADDER INFECTION

See Cholecystitis

GALL STONES

Key   Barberry, Corydalis, Dandelion Leaf, Dandelion Root, Fringe Tree, Globe Artichoke, Greater Celandine, Peppermint, St Mary's Thistle

GANGRENE

Key   Echinacea Root, Ginkgo, Gotu Kola, Grape Seed

GASTRIC ACID, LOW

See Hypochlorhydria

GASTRIC ULCER

See Ulcer, peptic

GASTRITIS

Key   Barberry (if involving Helicobacter), Chamomile, Fenugreek, Golden Seal (if involving Helicobacter), Licorice, Marshmallow Root, Meadowsweet, Peppermint, Propolis, Ribwort, Rosehips, Slippery Elm, Thyme (chronic)

Other   Fringe Tree, Sundew

GASTROINTESTINAL TRACT, BLEEDING

See also Bleeding, internal

Key   Agrimony, Cranesbill, Rhubarb Root, Tienchi Ginseng, Witch Hazel Leaf, Yarrow

Other   Meadowsweet, Nettle Leaf, Raspberry Leaf

GASTROINTESTINAL TRACT, INFLAMMATION

Key   Chamomile, Fenugreek, Marshmallow Root, Meadowsweet, Slippery Elm

GASTRO-OESOPHAGEAL REFLUX

Key   Chamomile, Cramp Bark, Gentian (low doses), Licorice, Marshmallow Root, Meadowsweet, Slippery Elm, Yarrow

GENITAL HERPES

See Herpes simplex

GINGIVITIS

Key   Adhatoda (topically), Baptisia, Echinacea Root (also topically), Myrrh (topically), Propolis (topically), Sage (topically), Thyme (topically)

GLANDS, LYMPH ENLARGED

Key   Baptisia, Blue Flag, Calendula, Clivers, Echinacea Root, Poke Root

GLANDULAR FEVER

See also Post-viral syndromes

Key   Andrographis, Echinacea Root, Elder Berry, Elder Flower, (all acute doses if in acute phase), St John's Wort, St Mary's Thistle

GLAUCOMA

Key   Bilberry, Coleus (topically/alcohol free)

GOUT

Key   Celery, Sarsparilla

Other   Boswellia, Burdock, Dandelion Leaf, Devil's Claw, Globe Artichoke, Gravel Root, Juniper

GRAVES' DISEASE

See Hyperthyroidism

GUMS, BLEEDING

See also Gingivitis

Key   Adhatoda (topically), Bilberry, Cranesbill (topically), Grape Seed

HAEMATURIA

See also Cystitis

Key   Gravel Root, Horsetail (acute doses), Rehmannia, Shepherd's Purse (acute doses), Tienchi Ginseng, Yarrow

HAEMOCHROMATOSIS

Key   Green Tea , Gymnema, St Mary's Thistle

HAEMORRHOIDS

Key   Agrimony, Bilberry, Butcher's Broom, Calendula (topically), Gotu Kola, Grape Seed, Horsechestnut, Prickly Ash, Senna Pods (to soften stool), Slippery Elm (to soften stool)

Other   Aloes Resin (to soften stool), Cascara (to soften stool)

HAEMORRHOIDS, TOPICALLY

Key   Agrimony, Calendula (if bleeding), Horsechestnut (if not bleeding), Witch Hazel Leaf

HALITOSIS

Key   Cloves, Myrrh, Propolis, Thyme (all topically)

HANGOVER, TO PREVENT

Key   Korean Ginseng, Rosemary, Schisandra, St Mary's Thistle, Turmeric

HASHIMOTO'S DISEASE

See Hypothyroidism

HAY FEVER

Key   Albizia, Baical Skullcap, Elder Flower, Eyebright, Garlic, Golden Rod, Golden Seal, Ground Ivy, Horseradish, Nettle Leaf, Ribwort, Tylophora

Other   Boswellia, Feverfew

HEADACHE, SINUS

See also Catarrh, sinus

Key   Elder Flower, Eyebright, Golden Seal, Horseradish, Peppermint, Ribwort

HEADACHE, TENSION

Key   California Poppy (acute doses), Corydalis (acute doses), Feverfew (high doses), Hawthorn, Hops, Jamaica Dogwood (acute doses), Lime Flowers, Passionflower, Rosemary, Valerian, Willow Bark, Wood Betony

Other   Cascara (if linked to constipation), Cramp Bark, Kava (acute doses), Lavender, Mexican Valerian, Pasque Flower, Peppermint (topically), Sage, Skullcap

HEALING, TO PROMOTE

Key   Bilberry, Dan Shen (fractures especially), Echinacea Root, Ginkgo, Gotu Kola (also topically), Grape Seed, Tienchi Ginseng (traumatic injuries)

HEARING LOSS, IDIOPATHIC

Key   Coleus, Dan Shen, Ginger, Ginkgo

HEART ATTACK, TO PREVENT

See also Atherosclerosis and Angina

Key   Coleus (antiplatelet action), Dan Shen, Garlic, Hawthorn, Terminalia arjuna

HEART FAILURE

See Cardiac failure

HEARTBURN

See Gastro-oesophageal reflux

HEAVY METAL BURDEN, TO REDUCE

Key   Garlic, St Mary's Thistle

HELICOBACTER

See Ulcer, peptic

HEPATITIS A

See also Infection, acute

Key   Andrographis (especially useful, acute doses), Bupleurum, Dan Shen, Echinacea Root (acute doses), Phyllanthus, St Mary's Thistle, St John's Wort (acute doses)

HEPATITIS B

See also Infection, chronic

Key   Andrographis, Astragalus, Bupleurum, Dan Shen, Echinacea Root, Fringe Tree, Phyllanthus, Schisandra, St Mary's Thistle, St John's Wort

HEPATITIS C

See also Infection, chronic

Key   Andrographis, Astragalus, Bupleurum, Dan Shen, Echinacea Root, Fringe Tree, Phyllanthus, Schisandra, St Mary's Thistle, St John's Wort

HEPATITIS, CHRONIC ACTIVE

See also Autoimmune disease

Key   Bupleurum, Dan Shen, Echinacea Root, Phyllanthus, Schisandra, St Mary's Thistle, St John's Wort

HERPES SIMPLEX

Key   Calendula (topically), Echinacea Root (acute doses), Licorice (topically), Lemon Balm (topically), Lomatium, Propolis (topically), St John's Wort (acute doses)

HERPES ZOSTER

See Shingles

HIRSUTISM

Key   Fennel (topically)

HIVES

See Urticaria

HOT FLUSHES/FLASHES

See Menopausal symptoms

HYPERCHOLESTEROLAEMIA

Key   Garlic, Globe Artichoke, Gymnema, Rhubarb Root, Tienchi Ginseng

Other   Albizia (possible benefit), Fenugreek (powdered seed), Green Tea, Polygonum multiflorum, Terminalia arjuna, Turmeric

HYPERGLYCAEMIA

See Diabetes

HYPERHYDROSIS

Key   Rehmannia, Sage, Zizyphus

HYPERTENSION

Key   Astragalus, Baical Skullcap, Coleus, Cramp Bark, Dan Shen, Dandelion Leaf, Garlic, Hawthorn, Lime Flowers, Mistletoe, Olive Leaf, Valerian

Other   Mexican Valerian, Yarrow, Zizyphus

HYPERTENSIVE RETINOPATHY

See also Hypertension

Key   Bilberry, Ginkgo, Grape Seed

HYPERTHYROIDISM

See also Autoimmune disease and Bowel flora

Key   Bugleweed, Motherwort (for cardiac symptoms)

HYPERTYRAMINAEMIA

Key   Barberry, Golden Seal

HYPOCHLORHYDRIA

Key   Angelica Root, Cayenne, Coleus, Gentian, Ginger, Wormwood

HYPOGLYCAEMIA

See Dysglycaemia

HYPOTENSION

Key   Ginkgo, Licorice, Prickly Ash, Rehmannia

HYPOTENSION, POSTURAL

Key   Astragalus, Ginkgo, Hawthorn, Horsechestnut, Korean Ginseng, Licorice

HYPOTHYROIDISM

See also Autoimmune disease and Bowel flora

Key   Bacopa, Bladderwrack, Coleus, Withania

IMMUNE DEFICIENCY, CHRONIC

Key   Astragalus, Cat's Claw, Echinacea Root, Korean Ginseng, Poke Root, Reishi, Rhodiola, Shiitake, Siberian Ginseng, Withania

IMMUNITY, POOR

Key   Andrographis, Astragalus, Cat's Claw, Echinacea Root, Reishi, Shiitake, Siberian Ginseng

Other   Korean Ginseng, Pau D'Arco, Poke Root, Sheep Sorrel, Withania

IMPOTENCE

Key   Damiana, Ginkgo, Korean Ginseng, Rhodiola, Shatavari, Tribulus Leaf, Withania

Other   Saw Palmetto, Siberian Ginseng

INCONTINENCE, URINARY

Key   Agrimony, Corn Silk, Crataeva, Gravel Root, Horsetail

INDIGESTION

See Dyspepsia

INFANTILE COLIC

See Colic, infantile

INFECTION, ACUTE

Key   Andrographis (acute doses), Baical Skullcap (especially respiratory and gastrointestinal, acute doses), Baptisia (especially respiratory), Cayenne, Echinacea Root (acute doses), Elder Flower (for fever), Ginger, Poke Root

INFECTION, CHRONIC

Key   Andrographis, Astragalus, Baptisia (especially respiratory), Cat's Claw, Echinacea Root, Reishi, Shiitake

INFECTION, GASTROINTESTINAL

See also Bowel flora and Dysentery

Key   Barberry (acute non-viral), Echinacea Root, Fenugreek, Garlic, Golden Seal (acute non-viral with diarrhoea), Propolis

Other   Ladies Mantle, Marshmallow Root, Slippery Elm

INFECTION, PREVENTION

Key   Andrographis, Astragalus (especially in depleted patients), Cat's Claw, Echinacea Root, Korean Ginseng, Reishi, Rhodiola, Shiitake, Siberian Ginseng, Withania

INFECTION, VIRAL

Key   Andrographis (acute doses), Echinacea Root (acute doses), Elder Berry (acute doses), St John's Wort (enveloped viruses), Thuja (all viruses)

INFERTILITY

See Fertility, to enhance

INFESTATION, WORMS

See Worms, intestinal

INFLUENZA

See also Infection, acute

Key   Andrographis, Baptisia, Boneset (if marked by severe myalgia), Echinacea Root, Elder Berry, Elder Flower, Elecampane, Garlic, Golden Rod, Lime Flowers, Lomatium, Mullein, Peppermint, Pleurisy Root, Propolis, Vervain, Yarrow (all acute doses)

Other   Bupleurum, Lemon Balm, Wormwood

INJURIES, INTERNAL TREATMENT

See Healing

INJURIES, TOPICALLY

See Wounds, topically

INSECT BITES

Key   Calendula (topically), Chickweed (topically), Comfrey (topically)

Other   Arnica (topically)

INSOMNIA, NON-RESTORATIVE SLEEP

Key   Bacopa, Licorice, Oats Green, Oats Seed, Rehmannia, Siberian Ginseng, Withania, Zizyphus

INSOMNIA, SLEEP MAINTENANCE

Key   Bacopa, California Poppy, Chaste Tree, Hops, Jamaica Dogwood, Kava, Lavender, Lemon Balm, Mexican Valerian, Oats Green, Oats Seed, Passionflower, Skullcap, St John's Wort, Valerian, Withania

INSOMNIA, SLEEP ONSET

Key   California Poppy, Corydalis, Hops, Jamaica Dogwood, Kava, Lavender, Lemon Balm, Lime Flowers, Mexican Valerian, Oats Green, Oats Seed, Passionflower, Polygala, St John's Wort, Valerian, Withania, Zizyphus

Other   Chamomile, Pasque Flower

INSULIN RESISTANCE

See also Metabolic Syndrome X

Key   Cinnamon, Goat's Rue, Gymnema, Korean Ginseng, St Mary's Thistle

INTERMITTENT CLAUDICATION

See Circulation, peripheral impaired

IRRITABILITY

Key   Lemon Balm, Mexican Valerian, Passionflower, Polygala, Skullcap, St John's Wort, Valerian, Vervain, Zizyphus

IRRITABLE BOWEL SYNDROME

Key   Chamomile, Corydalis, Cramp Bark Globe Artichoke, Greater Celandine, Marshmallow Root, Meadowsweet, Peppermint (especially essential oil), Skullcap, Slippery Elm, St John's Wort, Valerian

Other   Chaste Tree, Fennel, Fringe Tree, Ginger, Hops, Lavender, Lemon Balm

ITCHING

See Pruritis

JAUNDICE

See Hepatitis

JET LAG

See also Deep vein thrombosis

Key   Andrographis, Chaste Tree, Echinacea Root, Ginkgo, Kava, Rhodiola, Siberian Ginseng, St John's Wort, Valerian, Withania

KIDNEY STONES

Key   Bearberry, Crataeva, Golden Rod, Gravel Root, Hydrangea

Other   Clivers, Corn Silk, Couch Grass

LABOUR, TO ASSIST

See Pregnancy

LACTATION, DIFFICULT

Key   Fennel, Fenugreek, Goat's Rue, Shatavari, Vervain

Other   Aniseed, Chaste Tree (controversial)

LACTATION, TO INHIBIT

Key   Sage

Other   Peppermint

LARYNGITIS

Key   Cayenne (topically), Cloves (topically), Echinacea Root, Elder Flower, Euphorbia, Marshmallow Root (topically), Poke Root, Ribwort (topically), Sage (topically), Thyme

LATENT HYPERPROLACTINAEMIA

Key   Chaste Tree

LEUCORRHOEA

Key   False Unicorn, Ladies Mantle, Paeonia

LEUCORRHOEA AND VAGINITIS, AS A DOUCHE

Key   Bayberry, Beth Root, Cranesbill, Ladies Mantle

LEUKAEMIA

See Chronic lymphocytic leukaemia

LEUKOPAENIA

Key   Astragalus, Polygonum cuspidatum, Withania

LIBIDO, EXCESSIVE IN MEN

Key   Chaste Tree (higher doses), Hops

LIBIDO, TO ENHANCE

Key   Damiana, Korean Ginseng, Tribulus Leaf

LIVER CIRRHOSIS

Key   Dan Shen, Globe Artichoke, Gotu Kola, Grape Seed, Schisandra, St Mary's Thistle

LIVER DAMAGE

Key   Andrographis, Bupleurum, Dong Quai, Globe Artichoke, Schisandra, St Mary's Thistle

LIVER INSUFFICIENCY, DIGESTIVE

Key   Andrographis, Barberry, Blue Flag, Butternut, Bupleurum, Dandelion Leaf, Dandelion Root, Fringe Tree, Globe Artichoke, Greater Celandine, St Mary's Thistle

LIVER INSUFFICIENCY, PHASE I/II DETOXIFICATION

Key   Garlic, Green Tea, Rosemary, Schisandra, Turmeric

LOW GASTRIC ACID

See Hypochlorhydria

LUPUS

See also Autoimmune disease

Key   Astragalus, Boswellia, Bupleurum, Echinacea Root, Grape Seed, Hemidesmus, Qing Hao (high doses), Rehmannia, Siberian Ginseng, Tylophora

LYME DISEASE

See also Autoimmune disease and Infection, chronic

Key   Andrographis, Astragalus, Cat's Claw, Echinacea Root, Reishi

LYMPHADENOPATHY, LYMPHADENITIS

See Glands, lymph enlarged

LYMPHOEDEMA

Key   Butcher's Broom, Dandelion Leaf, Horsechestnut

MACULAR DEGENERATION

Key   Bilberry, Ginkgo, Grape Seed

MASTALGIA

Key   Blue Cohosh, Butcher's Broom, Chaste Tree, Evening Primrose Oil, Ginkgo

MASTITIS

Key   Echinacea Root (acute doses), Poke Root (also topically)

MEASLES

See also Infection, acute

Key   Andrographis, Echinacea Root, Elder Flower, Eyebright, St John's Wort (all acute doses)

MELASMA

Key   Bearberry (topically), Licorice (topically)

MEMORY, TO IMPROVE

Key   Bacopa (especially medium and long-term), Ginkgo (short-term), Korean Ginseng, Paeonia, Rhodiola, Rosemary, Sage, Schisandra, Siberian Ginseng

MENIERE'S DISEASE

Key   Ginkgo, Horsechestnut, Wood Betony

MENOPAUSAL SYMPTOMS

Key   Alfalfa, Black Cohosh, False Unicorn, Kava, Korean Ginseng, Ladies Mantle, Sage, Shatavari, St John's Wort, Tribulus Leaf, Wild Yam (oral use only)

Other   Chaste Tree (for pre-menstrual-like symptoms), Hawthorn, Hops, Oats Seed

MENORRHAGIA

See also Fibroids

Key   Beth Root (also topically), Chaste Tree, Cranesbill, Ladies Mantle, Paeonia, Shepherd's Purse (also topically), Tienchi Ginseng, Witch Hazel Leaf (topically), Yarrow

Other   False Unicorn, Golden Seal

MENSTRUAL IRREGULARITY

Key   Chaste Tree, Dong Quai, Paeonia

MENSTRUAL PAIN

See Dysmenorrhoea

MENTAL PERFORMANCE

See Cognitive performance

METABOLIC SYNDROME X

Key   Cinnamon (higher doses), Coleus, Gymnema, St Mary's Thistle

Other   Globe Artichoke, Goat's Rue, Licorice (for fat loss), Polygonum cuspidatum

METRORRHAGIA

Key   Beth Root, Chaste Tree, Cranesbill, Ladies Mantle, Rehmannia, Shepherd's Purse, Tienchi Ginseng

MIGRAINE HEADACHE

Key   Feverfew, Greater Celandine, Jamaica Dogwood, Willow Bark

Other   Lime Flowers, Paeonia, Valerian

MISCARRIAGE, REPEATED

Key   Black Haw, Chaste Tree, Cramp Bark, False Unicorn

MISCARRIAGE, THREATENED

Key   Black Haw, Chaste Tree, Cramp Bark, False Unicorn, Squaw Vine, True Unicorn, Wild Yam

MONONUCLEOSIS

See Glandular fever

MORNING SICKNESS

Key   Chen Pi, False Unicorn, Ginger, Peppermint, Raspberry Leaf (take from 2nd trimester)

MOTION SICKNESS

See Travel sickness

MOUTH ULCERS

See Ulcer, mouth

MULTIPLE SCLEROSIS

See also Autoimmune disease and Bowel flora

Key   Astragalus, Boswellia, Bupleurum, Echinacea Root (controversial), Ginkgo, Grape Seed, Hemidesmus, Rehmannia, St. John's Wort, Tylophora

MUMPS

Key   Andrographis, Echinacea Root, Poke Root

MUSCULAR TENSION

Key   Kava

MYALGIA

Key   Black Cohosh, Devil's Claw, Golden Seal, Meadowsweet, Tribulus

MYALGIA, TOPICALLY

Key   Arnica, Cayenne, Comfrey

MYOCARDIAL ISCHAEMIA

See Angina pectoris

NAILS, BRITTLE

Key   Gotu Kola, Horsetail, Nettle Leaf

NAPPY RASH

Key   Calendula (topically), Pau D'Arco (topically), Propolis (topically)

NAUSEA

Key   Bupleurum, Chen Pi, Cinnamon, Cloves, Fennel, Fringe Tree, Gentian, Ginger, Globe Artichoke, Golden Seal, Peppermint, St Mary's Thistle, Wormwood

Other   Barberry

NEPHRITIS

Key   Astragalus, Bilberry, Ginkgo, Gotu Kola, Golden Rod, Grape Seed, Rehmannia, Rhubarb Root, Sarsaparilla

NERVE DAMAGE

Key   Ginkgo, Gotu Kola, Grape Seed, St John's Wort

NERVOUS (SIMPLE) TACHYCARDIA

Key   Motherwort

NERVOUS DYSPEPSIA

Key   Chamomile, Damiana, Hops, Lavender, Lemon Balm, Mugwort, Valerian

NERVOUS EXHAUSTION

See Fatigue

NERVOUS TENSION

See Anxiety

NEURALGIA

See also Trigeminal neuralgia

Key   California Poppy (acute doses), Hops, Jamaica Dogwood (acute doses), St John's Wort (acute doses), Wood Betony

Other   Kava, Motherwort, Prickly Ash, Skullcap

NEURALGIA, TOPICALLY

Key   Cayenne, Peppermint

NEURASTHENIA

See Fatigue

NIGHT BLINDNESS

Key   Bilberry

NIGHT CRAMPS

Key   Butcher's Broom, Ginkgo, Gotu Kola, Horsechestnut, Kava, Valerian

NIGHT SWEATS

Key   Astragalus, Cat's Claw, Schisandra, Zizyphus

NOSE BLEED

See Epistaxis

OBESITY

See Weight loss, to assist

OEDEMA

Key   Boswellia (due to malignant brain tumours), Butcher's Broom, Dandelion Leaf, Horsechestnut

OEDEMA, PREMENSTRUAL

See Mastalgia

OESTROGEN, LOW

Key   False Unicorn, Korean Ginseng, Shatavari, Tribulus, Wild Yam

OESTROGEN, RELATIVE EXCESS

Key   Chaste Tree, Paeonia

OLIGOMENORRHOEA

Key   Chaste Tree

ORCHITIS

Key   Pasque Flower, Saw Palmetto

OSTEOARTHRITIS

Key   Arnica (topically), Black Cohosh (especially small joint), Boswellia, Cat's Claw, Cayenne (topically), Celery, Comfrey (topically), Devil's Claw, Ginger, Juniper, Nettle Leaf, Polygonum cuspidatum, Polygonum multiflorum, Prickly Ash, Rosehips (higher doses), Turmeric, Willow Bark, Withania

Other   Bladderwrack (in association with obesity), Garlic, Golden Rod, Gotu Kola, Horseradish (topically), Peppermint (topically), Rehmannia, Yellow Dock

OSTEOPENIA

Key   Coleus, Evening Primrose Oil, Gotu Kola

OTITIS MEDIA, INFECTIOUS

See also Common cold

Key   Andrographis, Echinacea Root, Elder Berry, Elder Flower, Eyebright, Pelargonium, Propolis, Ribwort

OTITIS MEDIA, SEROUS

See also Catarrh, nasopharyngeal

Key   Elder Flower, Eyebright, Golden Rod, Golden Seal, Ground Ivy, Ribwort

OVARIAN PAIN

Key   Blue Cohosh, False Unicorn, Motherwort, Pasque Flower, Wild Yam

OVARIAN CYST

Key   Chaste Tree (follicular), False Unicorn

OVULATION, ERRATIC

Key   Chaste Tree, Dong Quai, False Unicorn, Paeonia, Wild Yam

OVULATION, PAINFUL

See also Ovarian pain

Key   Chaste Tree

PAIN MANAGEMENT

See also Osteoarthritis, Neuralgia and Headache

Key   California Poppy (nerve generated pain/acute doses), Corydalis (visceral pain), Jamaica Dogwood (nerve generated pain/acute doses), Willow Bark (back pain)

PALPITATIONS

Key   Corydalis, Dan Shen, Dong Quai, Hawthorn, Lime Flowers, Motherwort, Passionflower, Polygala, Zizyphus

PANCREATITIS

Key   Dan Shen, Fringe Tree, Grape Seed, Rhubarb Root (acute)

PANIC ATTACKS

See also Anxiety

Key   California Poppy, Hops, Kava, Mexican Valerian, Valerian (all acute doses)

PARASITES, INTESTINAL

Key   Aniseed, Euphorbia (acute doses), Gentian (reduce infestation), Golden Seal, Myrrh (high doses for short periods), Pau D'Arco, Qing Hao, Wormwood

PARKINSON'S DISEASE

Key Ginkgo, Grape Seed, Rosemary, Turmeric

PELVIC INFLAMMATION, CHRONIC

Key Astragalus, Echinacea Root, False Unicorn, Saw Palmetto

PEPTIC ULCER

See Ulcer, peptic

PERTUSSIS

Key Aniseed, Echinacea Root, Elecampane, Euphorbia, Grindelia, Pleurisy Root, Sundew, Thyme, White Horehound, Wild Cherry (all acute doses)

PHARYNGITIS

Key Cloves (topically), Cranesbill (topically), Echinacea Root, Elder Flower, Eyebright, Fennel (topically), Golden Rod, Golden Seal, Ground Ivy, Kava (topically), Marshmallow Root (topically), Mullein, Myrrh (topically), Pelargonium (for acute), Poke Root, Raspberry Leaf (topically), Ribwort (also topically), Sage, Thyme (also topically)

Other Bayberry, Hyssop (topically as a gargle)

PHLEBITIS

See Thrombophlebitis

PHYSICAL PERFORMANCE

See Exercise

PILES

See Haemorrhoids

PLEURISY

See also Bronchitis, acute

Key Andrographis, Angelica Root, Echinacea Root, Elder Flower, Pelargonium, Pleurisy Root, Wild Cherry (all acute doses)

PNEUMONIA

See also Bronchitis, acute

Key Andrographis, Echinacea Root, Elecampane, Pleurisy Root, Wild Cherry (all acute doses)

Other Baptisia, Pelargonium

POLYCYSTIC OVARY SYNDROME

See also Insulin resistance

Key Black Cohosh, Chaste Tree, Gymnema, Licorice, Paeonia, Thuja, Tribulus Leaf

POLYMENORRHOEA

Key Chaste Tree

POST-PARTUM HAEMORRHAGE

Key Adhatoda, Beth Root, Black Haw, Golden Seal, Shepherd's Purse, Tienchi Ginseng (all acute doses)

POST-VIRAL SYNDROMES

See also Chronic fatigue syndrome

Key Astragalus, Korean Ginseng, Lomatium, Rhodiola, St John's Wort, Withania

Other Echinacea Root, Evening Primrose Oil, Reishi, Shiitake, Siberian Ginseng

PREGNANCY, FALSE LABOUR PAINS

Key Black Haw, Cramp Bark, Squaw Vine

PREGNANCY, NAUSEA

See Morning sickness

PREGNANCY, RESTLESS FOETUS

Key Baical Skullcap

PREGNANCY, TO PREPARE FOR LABOUR

Key Black Cohosh (in late pregnancy), Blue Cohosh (in late pregnancy), Cramp Bark (in late pregnancy), Raspberry Leaf (take from 2nd trimester), Squaw Vine

PREMENSTRUAL SYNDROME

Key Black Cohosh, Blue Cohosh, Butcher's Broom, Chaste Tree, Evening Primrose Oil, Skullcap, St John's Wort

PROGESTERONE DEFICIENCY

See Oestrogen, relative excess

PROSTATISM

Key Corydalis, Cramp Bark, Kava, Valerian

PROSTATITIS, ACUTE

See also Infection, acute

Key   Andrographis (acute doses) Bearberry (acute doses), Corn Silk (acute doses), Couch Grass (acute doses), Echinacea Root (acute doses), Gravel Root, Horsetail, Hydrangea

Other   Buchu (acute doses), Juniper (acute doses)

PROSTATITIS, CHRONIC

Key   Corn Silk, Couch Grass, Echinacea Root, Gravel Root, Horsetail, Hydrangea, Nettle Root, Saw Palmetto

Other   Buchu, Corydalis (as spasmolytic), Cramp Bark (as spasmolytic), Kava

PRURITUS

See also Skin disorders, chronic

Key   Ladies Mantle (vulvae, topically), Peppermint (topically)

PRURITUS, ANAL

See also Bowel flora

Key   Calendula (topically), Comfrey (topically), Grape Seed, Green Tea

PSORIASIS

See also Skin disorders, chronic

Key   Blue Flag, Burdock, Chickweed (topically), Clivers, Coleus, Comfrey (topically), Echinacea Root, Gotu Kola (also topically), Greater Celandine, Oregon Grape (also topically), Red Clover Flower, Sarsaparilla, Yellow Dock

Other   Boswellia

RADIOTHERAPY

See Cancer, during radiotherapy

RAYNAUD'S SYNDROME

Key   Cayenne, Cramp Bark, Evening Primrose Oil, Ginger, Ginkgo, Hawthorn, Prickly Ash

RECOVERY FROM DISEASE

See Convalescence

REPETITIVE STRAIN INJURY (RSI)

Key   Arnica (topically), Boswellia, Butcher's Broom, Cayenne (topically), Celery, Ginger, Ginkgo, Gotu Kola, Horsechestnut (also topically), St John's Wort, Turmeric, Willow Bark

RESTLESS LEGS SYNDROME

Key   Butcher's Broom, Ginkgo, Gotu Kola, Horsechestnut, Kava, Mexican Valerian, Prickly Ash, Valerian

RESTLESSNESS

See Anxiety

RETINAL BLOOD FLOW DISORDERS

Key   Bilberry, Ginkgo, Grape Seed

RETINAL DAMAGE

Key   Bilberry, Ginkgo, Gotu Kola, Grape Seed

RHEUMATISM

Key   Celery, Ginger, Juniper, Nettle Leaf, Sarsaparilla

Other   Burdock, Dandelion Root, Devil's Claw, Gravel Root, Meadowsweet, Prickly Ash, Yellow Dock

RHEUMATOID ARTHRITIS

See also Autoimmune disease and Bowel flora

Key   Black Cohosh, Boswellia, Cat's Claw, Cayenne (topically), Celery, Devil's Claw, Evening Primrose Oil, Feverfew, Ginger, Hemidesmus, Nettle Leaf, Polygonum cuspidatum, Rehmannia, Sarsaparilla, Turmeric, Tylophora, Willow Bark

Other   Burdock, Golden Rod, Wild Yam, Yellow Dock

RHINITIS, ALLERGIC

See Hay fever

ROSACEA

Key   Andrographis, Blue Flag, Burdock, Clivers, Echinacea Root, Golden Seal, Oregon Grape, Sarsaparilla

ROSS RIVER VIRUS

Key   Andrographis, Astragalus (for chronic), Cat's Claw (for chronic), Echinacea Root

SALPINGITIS

See Pelvic inflammation, chronic

SCIATICA

See Disc prolapse

SCLERODERMA

See also Autoimmune disease

Key   Dan Shen, Gotu Kola

SEBACEOUS CYSTS

Key   Calendula (internal)

SEIZURES

See Epilepsy

SENILE MACULAR DEGENERATION

See Macular degeneration

SHINGLES

Key   Andrographis, Cayenne (topically for post herpetic neuralgia), Echinacea Root, Licorice (topically), Lemon Balm (topically), Propolis (topically), St John's Wort

SINUSITIS, ACUTE

See also Common cold

Key   Andrographis, Echinacea Root, Elder Flower (acute doses), Eyebright, Garlic, Horseradish, Pelargonium, Ribwort, Thuja

SINUSITIS, ALLERGIC

See Hay fever

SINUSITIS, CHRONIC

Key   Andrographis, Echinacea Root, Elder Flower, Eyebright, Garlic, Golden Rod, Golden Seal, Ground Ivy, Horseradish, Propolis, Ribwort

SKIN ALLERGIES

See Dermatitis

SKIN DISORDERS, CHRONIC

Key   Black Walnut, Blue Flag, Burdock, Chickweed (topically), Clivers, Fringe Tree, Globe Artichoke, Hemidesmus, Oregon Grape, Poke Root, Red Clover Flower, Sarsaparilla, Turmeric (topically), Witch Hazel Leaf (topically), Yarrow (topically), Yellow Dock

Other   Dandelion Root

SMOKING, TO SUPPORT HEALTH

See also Bronchitis, chronic

Key   Andrographis, Echinacea Root, Grape Seed, Green Tea, Rosemary, Schisandra, Turmeric

SORE THROAT

See Pharyngitis

SPERM COUNT, LOW

See Fertility, male, to enhance

SPIDER VEINS

Key   Bilberry, Butcher's Broom, Grape Seed, Horsechestnut

SPLENIC ENLARGEMENT

Key   Blue Flag, Echinacea Root, Fringe Tree

SPORTS PERFORMANCE

See Exercise

SPRAINS

Key   Arnica (topically), Boswellia (acute doses), Comfrey (topically), Horsechestnut (topically)

STEROIDS, TO SUPPORT WITHDRAWAL FROM

Key   Licorice, Rehmannia

STOMATITIS

Key   Propolis (topically), Raspberry Leaf, Sage, Thyme (topically)

STRESS, EMOTIONAL

Key   California Poppy, Corydalis, Jamaica Dogwood, Kava, Mexican Valerian, Skullcap, St John's Wort, Valerian, Zizyphus

STRESS, PHYSICAL

Key   Korean Ginseng, Licorice, Rhodiola, Sarsaparilla, Schisandra, Siberian Ginseng, Tribulus Leaf, Withania

STROKE, RECOVERY AFTER

See also Dementia, vascular

Key   Bacopa, Ginkgo (recent onset), Grape
        Seed

SURGERY, PRE AND POST OPERATIVE

See also Healing

Key   Echinacea Root (post), Gotu Kola
        (post), St Mary's Thistle (pre and
        post)

SWEATING, EXCESSIVE

Key   Rehmannia, Sage, Zizyphus

SWEET CRAVING

Key   Gymnema, Licorice, Rehmannia

SYSTEMIC LUPUS ERYTHEMATOSUS

See Lupus

TACHYCARDIA

See also Arrhythmias

Key   Corydalis, Hawthorn, Mistletoe,
        Motherwort, Passionflower (nervous),
        Valerian

TEETHING

Key   Chamomile

TENNIS ELBOW

See herbs for Carpal Tunnel Syndrome

TESTICULAR ATROPHY

Key   Saw Palmetto, Tribulus

THROAT, SORE

See Pharyngitis

THROMBOCYTOPAENIA

See also Autoimmune disease

Key   Barberry

THROMBOPHLEBITIS

Key   Butcher's Broom, Gotu Kola,
        Horsechestnut

THROMBOSIS

See Deep vein thrombosis

THRUSH

See Candidiasis, vaginal

THYROTOXICOSIS

See Hyperthyroidism

TINEA

Key   Andrographis, Echinacea Root,
        Pau D'Arco (topically), Poke Root
        (topically), Stemona (topically),
        Thuja (topically)

TINNITUS

See also Anxiety

Key   Black Cohosh, Ginkgo (controversial),
        Polygonum multiflorum

TONSILLITIS

Key   Andrographis, Baptisia, Echinacea
        Root, Myrrh (topically), Pelargonium
        (for acute), Poke Root, Polygonum
        cuspidatum, Propolis, Raspberry Leaf
        (topically), Sage, Thyme (topically)

TOOTH DECAY

See Dental caries

TOOTHACHE

Key   California Poppy (acute doses),
        Cloves (topically), Jamaica Dogwood
        (acute doses), Kava (topically)

TRACHEITIS

See also Bronchitis, acute

Key   Mullein, Sundew, Wild Cherry

TRAVEL SICKNESS

Key   Chamomile, Ginger

TRIGEMINAL NEURALGIA

Key   California Poppy (acute doses), Grape
        Seed, Hops, Horsechestnut, Jamaica
        Dogwood, Kava, Passionflower,
        St John's Wort

TRIGLYCERIDES, ELEVATED

Key   Fenugreek (powdered seed), Garlic,
        Globe Artichoke, Gymnema, Rhubarb
        Root

TUBERCULOSIS

See also Infection, acute

Key   Pelargonium

ULCER, DIABETIC

Key   Calendula (topically), Echinacea Root
        (also topically), Ginkgo, Grape Seed,
        Gotu Kola

ULCER, MOUTH

Key   Baptisia, Calendula (topically), Chamomile (topically), Echinacea Root (liquid preferred), Licorice (also topically), Myrrh (topically), Propolis (also topically), Raspberry Leaf (topically)

ULCER, PEPTIC

Key   Barberry, Chamomile, Chickweed, Echinacea Root, Golden Seal, Gotu Kola, Licorice, Marshmallow Root, Meadowsweet, Propolis, Ribwort, Slippery Elm

Other   Fringe Tree, Mullein, Sundew

ULCER, PEPTIC FOR HELICOBACTER

Key   Andrographis, Cranberry, Echinacea Root, Garlic, Oregano, Rhubarb Root, Thyme, Turmeric

ULCER, VARICOSE

See Varicose ulcer

ULCERATIVE COLITIS

See also Autoimmune disease and Bowel flora

Key   Boswellia, Echinacea Root, Evening Primrose Oil, Golden Seal, Marshmallow Root, Propolis, Slippery Elm, St John's Wort

URETHRITIS

Key   Andrographis (acute doses), Bearberry (acute doses), Buchu (acute doses), Corn Silk, Couch Grass, Crataeva (acute doses), Echinacea Root (acute doses), Golden Rod, Horsetail, Hydrangea, Juniper (acute doses), Marshmallow Root, Meadowsweet

URINARY LITHIASIS

See Kidney stones

URINARY TRACT INFECTION

See Cystitis

URTICARIA

Key   Albizia, Baical Skullcap, Boswellia, Feverfew, Nettle Leaf, Rehmannia

UTERINE BLEEDING, DYSFUNCTIONAL

Key   Beth Root, Chaste Tree, False Unicorn, Nettle Leaf, Raspberry Leaf, Shepherd's Purse (also topically), Tienchi Ginseng

UTERINE PROLAPSE

Key   Astragalus, Blue Cohosh, Bupleurum (combined with Astragalus), False Unicorn, Raspberry Leaf

VARICOSE ULCER

Key   Andrographis, Butcher's Broom, Calendula (topically), Comfrey (topically), Echinacea Root (also topically), Ginkgo, Gotu Kola (also topically), Grape Seed, Horsechestnut, Marshmallow Root (topically), Propolis (topically), Ribwort (topically)

VARICOSE VEINS

Key   Agrimony (topically), Arnica (topically), Bilberry, Butcher's Broom, Calendula (topically), Gotu Kola (also topically), Grape Seed, Horsechestnut (also topically), Prickly Ash, Witch Hazel Leaf (topically)

VENOUS INSUFFICIENCY

Key   Agrimony, Arnica (topically), Bilberry (especially during pregnancy), Butcher's Broom, Gotu Kola, Grape Seed, Horsechestnut

VERTIGO

See Dizziness

VIRAL INFECTIONS

See Infections, viral

VISCERAL PAIN

Key   California Poppy, Corydalis, Cramp Bark, Jamaica Dogwood, Wild Yam

VISION, TO IMPROVE

Key   Bilberry, Ginkgo, Grape Seed, Schisandra

VISUAL FATIGUE

See Eye strain

VOMITING

See Nausea

WARTS

Key   Andrographis, Echinacea Root,
      Greater Celandine (topically), Thuja
      (also topically)

WEIGHT GAIN, TO ASSIST

Key   Codonopsis, Korean Ginseng,
      Rhodiola, Siberian Ginseng, Tribulus,
      Withania

WEIGHT LOSS, TO ASSIST

See also Metabolic syndrome X

Key   Bladderwrack (for poor thyroid
      activity), Cayenne, Coleus, Globe
      Artichoke, Green Tea, Gymnema

Other Blue Flag, Fennel (possibly), Goat's
      Rue, Licorice (for fat loss), Tienchi
      Ginseng

WHOOPING COUGH

See Pertussis

WORMS, INTESTINAL

Key   Andrographis (acute doses), Black
      Walnut, Cloves, Garlic, Myrrh (high
      doses for short periods), Stemona,
      Wormwood (acute doses)

Other Euphorbia (acute doses), Gentian (to
      reduce reinfestation), Mugwort

WOUNDS

See Healing, to promote

WOUNDS, TOPICALLY

Key   Calendula, Chamomile, Chickweed,
      Comfrey, Cranesbill, Echinacea Root,
      Golden Seal, Horsetail, Mullein,
      Myrrh, Propolis, St John's Wort
      (infused oil), Witch Hazel Leaf

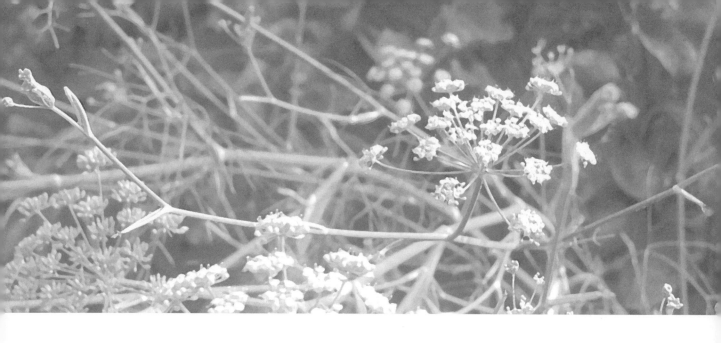

Treatment Protocols

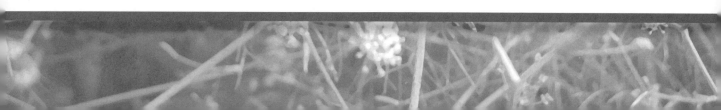

EXAMPLE LIQUID FORMULATION

Chaste Tree	1:2	15 mL
Calendula	1:2	20 mL
Burdock	1:2	20 mL
Baical Skullcap	1:2	20 mL
Poke Root	1:5	5 mL
Echinacea Root blend	1:2	30 mL
		110 mL

Dose: 5 mL with water 3 times a day or 8 mL twice a day

EXAMPLE TABLET/SINGLE LIQUID PROTOCOL

Core Treatment

Skin/Elimination Support (4 tablets per day)

AND

Chaste Tree (2 to 4 tablets per day on rising)

AND

Echinacea Formula (2 tablets once a day)

Additional Treatments (as required)

- Golden Seal or High Allicin Releasing Garlic (2 to 3 tablets of either per day) in stubborn cases, especially those marked by lesions filled with pus.
- Topical treatment with a tea tree oil or Calendula cream or liquid.
- Herbal Thyroid Support (3 to 4 tablets per day for the large tablets or 6 to 9 per day for the small tablets) if thyroid function is low.

Backup Treatment

Glucose Metabolism Support (2 to 3 tablets per day) instead of the Skin/Elimination Support in the above Core Treatment

EXAMPLE LIQUID FORMULATION

Echinacea Root blend	1:2	25 mL
Pleurisy Root	1:2	20 mL
Ginger	1:2	5 mL
Elecampane	1:2	20 mL
Licorice	1:1	15 mL
Fennel	1:2	20 mL
		105 mL

Dose: 5 mL with 40 mL warm water 5 to 6 times a day or 8 mL 3 to 4 times a day

EXAMPLE TABLET/SINGLE LIQUID PROTOCOL

Core Treatment

Short Term Lower Respiratory Support (5 to 6 tablets per day)

AND

Short Term Immune Support (4 to 6 tablets per day)

Additional Treatments (as required)

- Echinacea Formula (3 tablets per day) for additional immune support.
- Golden Seal (3 tablets per day) if there is excessive production of purulent mucus (but generally not in the febrile phase).
- Marshmallow Root 1:5 glycetract (4 mL as often as required, taken undiluted) to soothe a dry, unproductive cough or a chronic cough which persists once the infection is over.

Backup Treatment

High Allicin Releasing Garlic (3 tablets per day)

AND

Echinacea Formula (4 tablets per day)

EXAMPLE LIQUID FORMULATIONS

Morning and Day Formula

Paeonia	1:2	20 mL
Ginkgo	2:1	20 mL
Bacopa	1:2	30 mL
St John's Wort	1:2	25 mL
Korean Ginseng	1:2	15 mL
		110 mL

Dose: 8 mL with water twice a day

Evening Formula

Valerian	1:2	25 mL
Passionflower	1:2	25 mL
Skullcap	1:2	25 mL
Chamomile	1:2	25 mL
		100 mL

Dose: 8 mL with water before dinner and again one hour before bedtime

Note: These are adult doses. For children's doses use the calculation provided in the How to Use section. Some ADHD children may be aggravated by the evening treatment, in which case it should not be used

EXAMPLE TABLET/SINGLE LIQUID PROTOCOL

Core Treatment

Morning and Day

Memory/Brain Tonic (4 tablets per day)

AND

Ginkgo (3 tablets or 3 mL of 2:1 liquid with water per day)

AND

Stress Control (4 tablets per day)

Evenings

Sleep/Anxiety Support (3 to 4 tablets per day)

Additional Treatments (as required)

- Chamomile 1:2 (4 mL with water) in the evening for additional calming effect.
- Skullcap 1:2 (4 mL with water once or twice during the day) for the angry, aggressive child.
- Paeonia 1:2 (4 mL with water once or twice during the day) instead of the Memory/Brain Tonic or the Ginkgo for cognition enhancement.

Note: These are adult doses. For children's doses use the calculations provided. Some ADHD children may be aggravated by the evening treatments, in which case they should not be used

ADRENAL DEPLETION

EXAMPLE LIQUID FORMULATION

Licorice	1:1	15 mL
Rehmannia	1:2	25 mL
Withania	1:1	30 mL
Siberian Ginseng	1:2	30 mL
		100 mL

Dose: 8 mL with water twice a day

EXAMPLE TABLET/SINGLE LIQUID PROTOCOL

Core Treatment

Rehmannia 1:2 (4 mL with water per day)

AND

Stress Control (3 to 4 tablets per day) if the patient sleeps soundly OR Stress Adapt (3 to 4 tablets per day) if the patient tends to sleep poorly. In extreme cases of depletion these two products can be combined

PROTOCOLS

Additional Treatments (as required)

- Nervous System Tonic (3 to 4 tablets per day) if emotional stress and a depleted nervous system are present.
- Long Term Immune Support (3 to 4 tablets per day), switching to Short Term Immune Support (6 to 8 tablets per day) during infections, if recurrent infections are a feature.
- Licorice 1:1 (3 mL per day) if additional adrenal support is required, especially if the patient has low blood pressure. (Caution with additional Licorice liquid if Stress Control is already being taken.)

ALLERGIC RHINITIS

See Hayfever

ALZHEIMER'S DISEASE

EXAMPLE LIQUID FORMULATION

Korean Ginseng	1:2	15 mL
Ginkgo	2:1	30 mL
Paeonia	1:2	25 mL
Bacopa	1:2	30 mL
		100 mL

Dose: 5 mL with water 3 times a day or 8 mL twice a day

EXAMPLE TABLET/SINGLE LIQUID PROTOCOL

Core Treatment

Ginkgo (4 to 6 tablets or 4 to 6 mL of 2:1 liquid with water per day)

AND

Memory/Brain Tonic (3 to 4 tablets per day)

Additional Treatments (as required)

- Herbal Antioxidant (2 tablets per day) as an antioxidant support to prevent further deterioration.

- Paeonia 1:2 (5 mL with water per day) AND/OR Korean Ginseng 1:2 (3 mL with water per day) AND/OR Sage 1:2 (5 mL with water per day) for additional effects on cognition enhancement.
- St John's Wort (3 to 4 tablets per day) for associated depression.
- Sleep/Anxiety Support (3 to 4 tablets per day) for associated anxiety or insomnia.

Prevention

Ginkgo (2 to 3 tablets or 2 to 3 mL of 2:1 liquid with water per day)

AND

Herbal Antioxidant (2 tablets per day)

AND

Bilberry (2 tablets per day) and blueberries in the diet

ANXIETY

EXAMPLE LIQUID FORMULATION

Passionflower	1:2	30 mL
Skullcap	1:2	20 mL
Valerian	1:2	25 mL
Bacopa	1:2	25 mL
		100 mL

Dose: 5 mL with water 3 times a day or 8 mL twice a day

EXAMPLE TABLET/SINGLE LIQUID PROTOCOL

Core Treatment

Sleep/Anxiety Support or Anxiety Support (3 to 4 tablets per day)

Additional Treatments (as required)

- Nervous System Tonic (3 to 4 tablets per day) if low mood and nervous depletion is present.
- Stress Control (3 to 4 tablets per day) for any associated adrenal depletion.

- Smooth Muscle Relaxant (3 to 4 tablets per day) if the anxiety causes spasm or tension in visceral organs.
- Extra Sleep/Anxiety Support or Anxiety Support (2 tablets before bed) if insomnia is also present.

ASTHMA

EXAMPLE LIQUID FORMULATIONS

For both symptomatic treatment and dealing with underlying factors where concurrent sinusitis is involved.

Baical Skullcap	1:2	30 mL
Ginkgo	2:1	25 mL
Eyebright	1:2	15 mL
Echinacea Root blend	1:2	30 mL
		100 mL

Dose: 5 mL with water 3 to 4 times a day or 8 mL 2 to 3 times per day

For night cough/gastro-oesophageal reflux

Licorice	1:1	15 mL
Meadowsweet	1:2	20 mL
Marshmallow Root glycetract	1:5	65 mL
		100 mL

Dose: 3 to 5 mL undiluted as required up to 6 times a day

EXAMPLE TABLET/SINGLE LIQUID PROTOCOL

Core Treatment

Chronic Lung Support (3 to 4 tablets per day)

AND

Echinacea Formula (2 tablets per day) especially for late onset asthma

AND

Upper Respiratory Tract Support (3 to 4 tablets per day) if sinusitis or sinus allergy is present or otherwise one of the options below.

Additional Treatments (as required)

- Clear Lung Formula (3 to 4 tablets per day) instead of Upper Respiratory Tract Support if there is no evidence of sinus involvement and/or the patient has highly congested lungs (so-called bronchial asthma).
- Boswellia Combination (2 to 3 tablets per day) to control chronic inflammation (especially for intrinsic or exercise-induced asthma).
- Upper Digestive Formula (1 tablet before each meal) if there is evidence of functional hypochlorhydria.
- Marshmallow Root 1:5 glycetract (sipped undiluted as required) for gastro-oesophageal reflux or night cough.
- Allergy Support (3 to 4 tablets per day) if there is a strong allergic component.

BENIGN PROSTATIC HYPERPLASIA

EXAMPLE LIQUID FORMULATIONS

Saw Palmetto	1:2	35 mL
Nettle Root	1:2	25 mL
Crataeva	1:2	40 mL
		100 mL

Dose: 5 mL with water 3 times a day or 8 mL twice a day

Where an element of prostatism is present

Corydalis	1:2	20 mL
Saw Palmetto	1:2	35 mL
Nettle Root	1:2	25 mL
Cramp Bark	1:2	20 mL
		100 mL

Dose: 5 mL with water 3 times a day or 8 mL twice a day

EXAMPLE TABLET/SINGLE LIQUID PROTOCOL

Core Treatment

Prostate Support (3 to 4 capsules per day)

Additional Treatments (as required)

- Smooth Muscle Relaxant (3 to 4 tablets per day) if prostatism is also present.
- Korean Ginseng 1:2 (2 mL with water once a day) if the patient also complains of impotence.
- Urinary Tract Support (3 to 4 tablets per day) for low grade infection and chronic urinary retention. Add Short Term Immune Support (6 tablets per day) during acute infections.

Backup Treatment

Sometimes the main cause of symptoms is prostatism. If this is the case the above Core Treatment may not be effective and the protocol given below should be followed:

Smooth Muscle Relaxant (3 to 4 tablets per day)

AND

Sleep/Anxiety Support (3 to 4 tablets per day)

BOWEL FLORA DYSBIOSIS

EXAMPLE TABLET/SINGLE LIQUID PROTOCOL

Core Treatment

For two consecutive days of the week:

High Allicin Releasing Garlic (3 to 4 tablets per day)

AND

Bowel Flora Complex (4 to 6 tablets per day)

For the other five days of the week:

Slippery Elm (3 capsules with water 3 times a day)

AND

Herbal Antioxidant (2 tablets per day)

Additional Treatments (as required)

- Upper Digestive Formula (one tablet sucked for 30 to 60 seconds before each meal throughout the week) to improve the gastric acid barrier, digestive function in general and immune function.
- Echinacea Formula (3 tablets per day throughout the week) to improve immune function.

- Golden Seal (4 tablets per day, 2 plus 2, on the same two days as the other antimicrobial herbs) for extra antimicrobial activity.

CANCER, ADJUNCTIVE SUPPORT

EXAMPLE LIQUID FORMULATION

Astragalus	1:2	25 mL
Cat's Claw	1:2	25 mL
Korean Ginseng	1:2	15 mL
Siberian Ginseng	1:2	25 mL
Poke Root	1:5	2.5 mL
Licorice	1:1	10 mL
		102.5 mL

Dose: 7 mL with water 3 times a day

EXAMPLE TABLET/SINGLE LIQUID PROTOCOL

Core Treatment

Sheep Sorrel Formula (4 tablets per day)

AND

Cat's Claw Immune Formula (4 tablets per day)

Additional Treatments (as required)

- Mushroom Immune Formula (4 tablets per day) and/or Echinacea Formula (3 tablets per day) and/or Long Term Immune Support (4 tablets per day) where additional immune support is required.
- Herbal Antioxidant (2 tablets per day) and Liver Detox Assist (3 tablets per day) to support hepatic detoxification activity and provide antioxidant activity, but not during chemotherapy or radiotherapy.
- Anti-inflammatory herbs, in particular following surgery to reduce the risk of metastasis, especially Ginkgo (6 tablets per day or 6 mL of 2:1 liquid) and Boswellia Combination (4 tablets per day).
- California Poppy 1:2 (5 mL with water 1 to 4 times a day) for pain management.

- Liver Protection Formula (3 tablets per day) if there is a secondary liver tumour.

CANCER, DURING CHEMOTHERAPY

EXAMPLE LIQUID FORMULATION

Korean Ginseng	1:2	15 mL
Siberian Ginseng	1:2	30 mL
Withania	1:1	30 mL
Astragalus	1:2	30 mL
		105 mL

Dose: 8 mL with water 2 to 3 times a day
Works best in combination with Liver Protection Formula
(3 tablets per day)

EXAMPLE TABLET/SINGLE LIQUID PROTOCOL

Core Treatment

Liver Protection Formula (3 tablets per day)
AND
Long Term Immune Support (4 to 6 tablets per day)
AND
Mushroom Immune Formula (4 tablets per day)

Additional Treatment (as required)

- Stress Control (4 tablets per day) to support white cell count.
- Extra Stress Adapt (2 to 3 tablets per day) to counter toxic effects.
- Codonopsis 1:2 (5 mL with water 1 to 2 times a day) if red blood cell count drops too low.

CANCER, DURING RADIOTHERAPY

EXAMPLE LIQUID FORMULATION

Korean Ginseng	1:2	15 mL
Siberian Ginseng	1:2	30 mL
Withania	1:1	30 mL
Astragalus	1:2	30 mL
		105 mL

Dose: 8 mL with water 2 to 3 times a day

EXAMPLE TABLET/SINGLE LIQUID PROTOCOL

Core Treatment

Stress Adapt (4 tablets per day)
AND
Long Term Immune Support (4 to 6 tablets per day)
AND
Mushroom Immune Formula (4 tablets per day)

Additional Treatment (as required)

- Stress Control (4 tablets per day) to support white cell count.
- Codonopsis 1:2 (5 mL with water 1 to 2 times a day) if red blood cell count drops too low.
- Herbal Antioxidant (2 tablets per day) for antioxidant activity after the radiotherapy course is completed.
- Korean Ginseng 1:2 (3 mL with water 1 to 2 times a day) if energy is greatly depleted by the radiotherapy.

CHRONIC BRONCHITIS

EXAMPLE LIQUID FORMULATIONS

Immune formula (mainly)

Echinacea Root Blend	1:2	35 mL
Astragalus	1:2	25 mL
Mullein	1:2	20 mL
Withania	1:1	20 mL
		100 mL

Dose: 5 mL with water 3 times per day or 8 mL twice a day

Lung formula

Licorice	1:1	15 mL
Elecampane	1:2	20 mL
Ginger	1:2	10 mL
Fennel	1:2	15 mL
Thyme	1:2	20 mL
Grindelia	1:2	20 mL
		100 mL

Dose: 5 mL with water 3 times a day or 8 mL twice a day

Demulcent and antitussive formula

Marshmallow Root glycetract	1:5	80 mL
Licorice (high in glycyrrhizin)	1:1	20 mL
		100 mL

Dose: 4 mL sipped undiluted (that is no water is added) as required up to 4 times a day

EXAMPLE TABLET/SINGLE LIQUID PROTOCOL

Core Treatment

Clear Lung Formula (3 to 5 tablets per day)
AND
High Allicin Releasing Garlic (2 tablets per day)
AND
Echinacea Formula (2 to 3 tablets per day)

Additional Treatments (as required)

- Short Term Immune Support (6 tablets per day) and Short Term Lower Respiratory Support (6 tablets per day) replacing the Clear Lung Formula and Echinacea Formula during acute lung infections.
- Golden Seal (2 to 4 tablets per day) if the mucus coughed up is green/yellow and excessive.

- The demulcent and antitussive liquid formula above (or just Marshmallow Root 1:5 glycetract) if there is excessive and debilitating coughing at night.
- Herbal Antioxidant (2 tablets per day) if emphysema is predominant.
- Hawthorn (3 tablets per day) and Ginkgo (3 tablets per day) for blue bloaters.

Backup Treatment

Chronic Lung Support (3 to 5 tablets per day) instead of the Clear Lung Formula above

CHRONIC FATIGUE SYNDROME

EXAMPLE LIQUID FORMULATIONS

Korean Ginseng	1:2	10 mL
Withania	1:1	35 mL
St John's Wort	1:2	15 mL
Ginkgo	2:1	20 mL
Astragalus	1:2	30 mL
		110 mL

Dose: 5 mL with water 3 times a day or 8 mL twice a day

ALTERNATIVE EXAMPLE FORMULATION

Siberian Ginseng	1:2	30 mL
Rhodiola	2:1	40 mL
Codonopsis	1:2	30 mL
		100 mL

Dose: 5 mL with water 3 times a day or 8 mL twice a day

EXAMPLE TABLET/SINGLE LIQUID PROTOCOL

Core Treatment

Nervous System Tonic (4 tablets per day)
AND
Long Term Immune Support (4 tablets per day) switching to Short Term Immune Support (4 to 6 tablets per day) during acute infections

AND

Echinacea Formula (2 to 3 tablets per day)

Additional Treatments (as required)

- Stress Control (3 to 4 tablets per day) or Stress Adapt (2 to 3 tablets per day) to provide extra tonic activity.
- Ginkgo (3 to 4 tablets or 3 to 4 mL of 2:1 liquid with water per day) or Memory/Brain Tonic (3 to 4 tablets per day) for poor concentration and mental fatigue.
- Anxiety Support (3 tablets before bed) or Sleep/Anxiety Support (3 tablets before bed) to improve sleep quality.
- Boswellia Combination (3 to 4 tablets per day) if aches and pains are a feature.
- Autoimmune Formula (3 to 4 tablets per day) for adrenal tonic activity and to balance a dysregulated immune response.
- St John's Wort (3 to 4 tablets per day) instead of the Nervous System Tonic if depression is a marked feature or if there is a tendency to infection with enveloped viruses.
- Hawthorn for the autonomic imbalance and circulatory abnormalities (2 tablets per day) and Herbal Thyroid Support (3 tablets per day for the large tablets or 6 per day for the small tablets) if thyroid function is compromised.

Backup Treatments

Cat's Claw Immune Formula (3 to 4 tablets per day)

AND

Mushroom Immune Formula (3 to 4 tablets per day)

AND

Stress Control (3 to 4 tablets per day)

plus any of the above treatments as required

COMMON COLD

EXAMPLE LIQUID FORMULATION

Echinacea Root blend	1:2	35 mL
Ginger	1:2	5 mL
Lime Flowers	1:2	20 mL
Eyebright	1:2	20 mL
Elder Flowers	1:2	20 mL
		100 mL

Dose: 5 mL with 40 mL hot water 5 to 6 times a day

EXAMPLE TABLET/SINGLE LIQUID PROTOCOL

Core Treatment

Short Term Immune Support (4 to 8 tablets per day)

Additional Treatments (as required)

- Echinacea Formula (3 tablets per day) for additional immune support.
- Golden Seal (3 tablets per day) if there is a thick yellowish/green discharge.

Backup Treatment

Echinacea Formula (4 tablets per day)

AND

High Allicin Releasing Garlic (3 tablets per day)

CONCEPTION, DIFFICULTY WITH

See Infertility, female and male

CROHN'S DISEASE

EXAMPLE LIQUID FORMULATION

Echinacea Root blend	1:2	30 mL
Chamomile	1:2	20 mL
Rehmannia	1:2	20 mL
Bupleurum	1:2	20 mL
Licorice	1:1	15 mL
		105 mL

Dose: 5 mL with water 3 times a day or 8 mL twice a day
For best results combine with Boswellia Combination tablets and the Bowel flora dysbiosis protocol

EXAMPLE TABLET/SINGLE LIQUID PROTOCOL

Core Treatment

Echinacea Formula (3 tablets per day)

AND

Boswellia Combination (4 tablets per day)

AND

Bowel flora dysbiosis protocol

Additional Treatments (as required)

- Smooth Muscle Relaxant (3 to 4 tablets per day) for gut spasm and pain.
- Autoimmune Formula (3 to 4 tablets per day) for additional anti-inflammatory activity.
- High Allicin Releasing Garlic (2 tablets per day) or Golden Seal (3 to 4 tablets per day) for antimycobacterial activity (as an alternative to the bowel flora dysbiosis protocol).
- Chamomile 1:2 (high in bisabolol) (4 mL with water once a day) for gut inflammation and spasm.

CYSTITIS AND CYSTITIS, RECURRENT

EXAMPLE LIQUID FORMULATION

Echinacea Root blend	1:2	35 mL
Buchu	1:2	20 mL
Licorice	1:1	15 mL
Crataeva	1:2	30 mL
		100 mL

Dose: 5 mL with water 4 to 6 times a day for acute outbreaks of cystitis and 3 times a day to prevent recurrent cystitis

EXAMPLE TABLET/SINGLE LIQUID PROTOCOL

Core Treatment

For acute cystitis:

Short Term Immune Support (6 tablets per day)

AND

Urinary Tract Support (4 to 6 tablets per day)

To prevent recurrent cystitis:

Echinacea Formula (2 to 3 tablets per day)

AND

Urinary Tract Support (4 tablets per day)

Additional Treatment (as required)

- Long Term Immune Support (3 to 4 tablets per day) in patients with chronic immune debility. (Switch to Short Term Immune Support as above during acute infections.)

DEPRESSION

EXAMPLE LIQUID FORMULATION

Valerian	1:2	20 mL
St John's Wort	1:2	25 mL
Skullcap	1:2	20 mL
Schisandra	1:2	20 mL
Licorice	1:1	15 mL
		100 mL

Dose: 5 mL with water 3 times a day or 8 mL twice a day

EXAMPLE TABLET/SINGLE LIQUID PROTOCOL

Core Treatment

St John's Wort (3 to 4 tablets per day)

Additional Treatments (as required)

- Sleep/Anxiety Support (3 to 4 tablets per day) or Anxiety Support if there is associated anxiety. If sleep onset insomnia is a feature, also recommend before bed (in this case the dose becomes one tablet twice a day and 2 to 3 tablets before bed).
- Rehmannia 1:2 (4 mL with water per day) OR Licorice 1:1 (3 mL with water per day) to support the adrenal glands.
- Stress Adapt (3 to 4 tablets per day) OR Stress Control (3 to 4 tablets per day) if the patient is stressed, low in energy and run down to support the hypothalamic-pituitary-adrenal axis.
- Ginkgo (3 to 4 tablets per day) if the depression is linked to low blood pressure or cerebral ischaemia, especially indicated in an elderly patient.

Backup Treatment

- Nervous System Tonic (4 tablets per day) instead of, or in addition to, the St John's Wort. In the latter case reduce the St John's Wort tablets to 2 per day.

DERMATITIS (ECZEMA)

EXAMPLE LIQUID FORMULATIONS

For a child weighing 20 kg (44 lbs)

Echinacea Root blend	1:2	50 mL
Baical Skullcap	1:2	25 mL
Nettle Leaf	1:2	25 mL
		100 mL

Dose: 3 mL with water twice a day

For an adult

Astragalus	1:2	25 mL
Nettle Leaf	1:2	25 mL
Gotu Kola	1:2	20 mL
Feverfew	1:5	10 mL
Bupleurum	1:2	20 mL
		100 mL

Dose: 5 mL with water 3 times a day or 8 mL twice a day

EXAMPLE TABLET/SINGLE LIQUID PROTOCOL

Note: The doses given below represent adult doses. For children's doses use the calculation provided in the How to Use section.

Core Treatment

Echinacea Formula (2 tablets per day)

AND

Skin/Elimination Support (4 tablets per day)

AND

Allergy Support (3 to 4 tablets per day)

Additional Treatments (as required)

- Nettle Leaf 1:2 (4 mL with water per day) for additional anti-inflammatory and antiallergic activity.
- Upper Digestive Formula (1 tablet sucked for 30 to 60 seconds before each meal) if there is evidence of functional hypochlorhydria.
- Liver Detox Assist (3 to 4 tablets per day) if it is assessed that hepatic detoxification processes require boosting.
- Autoimmune Formula (3 to 4 tablets a day) as a long-term treatment to rebalance T-lymphocyte responses and provide anti-inflammatory effects.
- Evening Primrose Oil (3 capsules per day) for anti-inflammatory activity and to help correct any imbalance in essential fatty acid metabolism.

- Topical treatment with anti-inflammatory herbs such as Calendula, Licorice (high glycyrrhizin preparations), Gotu Kola or Chamomile (high in bisabolol) and antiseptic herbs such as Calendula, Myrrh or Golden Seal.

DIABETES, TYPE 2

EXAMPLE LIQUID FORMULATION

Licorice	1:1	15 mL
Baical Skullcap	1:2	25 mL
Goat's Rue	1:2	30 mL
Korean Ginseng	1:2	20 mL
Cinnamon (Cassia)	1:2	20 mL
		110 mL

Dose: 8 mL with water twice a day

EXAMPLE TABLET/SINGLE LIQUID PROTOCOL

Core Treatment

Glucose Metabolism Support (one tablet before each meal) AND

Liver Protection Formula (one tablet before each meal)

Additional Treatments (as required)

- Bilberry (4 tablets per day) for diabetic retinopathy.
- Bilberry (4 tablets per day) and Ginkgo (3 to 4 tablets per day) for associated microvascular problems such as nephropathy and neuropathy and/or Gotu Kola 1:1 (4 mL per day with water).
- Herbal Antioxidant (2 tablets per day) for antioxidant activity to help prevent diabetic complications.
- Licorice 1:1 (3 mL with water per day) and/or Baical Skullcap 1:2 (5 mL with water per day) to prevent long-term complications.
- Evening Primrose Oil (3 to 4 capsules per day) for diabetic neuropathy.

Backup Treatment

Korean Ginseng 1:2 (3 mL with water per day) instead of or in addition to the Liver Protection Formula in the Core Treatment

DIGESTIVE FUNCTION, TO IMPROVE

EXAMPLE LIQUID FORMULATION

Gentian	1:2	10 mL
Cinnamon	1:2	25 mL
Coleus	1:1	40 mL
Ginger	1:2	25 mL
		100 mL

Dose: 20 to 40 drops (about 0.5 to 1.0 mL) with water 20 minutes before meals

EXAMPLE TABLET/SINGLE LIQUID PROTOCOL

Core Treatment

Upper Digestive Formula (1 tablet 15 to 20 minutes before each meal, sucked for 30 to 60 seconds before swallowing)

Additional Treatments (as required)

- Liver/Biliary Tonic (1 tablet before each meal) if fat intolerance or other signs of liver stagnation are predominant.
- Liver Protection Formula (2 to 3 tablets per day) if there is evidence or a history of liver damage.

DYSGLYCAEMIA

EXAMPLE LIQUID FORMULATION

Rehmannia	1:2	30 mL
Licorice	1:1	15 mL
Gymnema	1:1	10 mL
Schisandra	1:2	25 mL
Siberian Ginseng	1:2	25 mL
		105 mL

Dose: 5 mL with water 3 times a day before meals or 8 mL twice a day

EXAMPLE TABLET/SINGLE LIQUID PROTOCOL

Core Treatment

Licorice 1:1 (3 mL with water per day) and/or Rehmannia 1:2 (4 mL with water per day)

AND

Glucose Metabolism Support (½ to 2 tablets per day)

Additional Treatments (as required)

- Stress Control (2 to 3 tablets per day) or Stress Adapt (2 to 3 tablets per day) if the hypoglycaemia is aggravated by stress. Stop the Licorice liquid and switch to Rehmannia liquid if Stress Control is prescribed.
- Liver Detox Assist (2 to 3 tablets per day) to support liver function if there is evidence of or a history of poor detoxifying capacity.
- Ginkgo (3 tablets per day or 3 mL of 2:1 liquid per day with water) if poor blood supply to the brain is an aggravating factor.

DYSMENORRHOEA, SPASMODIC

EXAMPLE LIQUID FORMULATIONS

For the Painful Period

About one week before the period is due, start the following herbal formulation:

California Poppy	1:2	25 mL
Wild Yam	1:2	30 mL
Cramp Bark	1:2	35 mL
Ginger	1:2	10 mL
		100 mL

Commence with a dose of 5 mL with water twice a day. Then just before menstruation, increase to 5 mL with water six times a day and stop treatment when pain has gone

Long-term Treatment

Not all women experience dysmenorrhoea. Hence it is not an inevitable consequence of menstruation. If the patient desires to treat the underlying condition, an additional long-term hormonal-balancing formula can be tried. Also in more severe cases of spasmodic dysmenorrhoea, this or similar hormonal-balancing treatments throughout the cycle are an essential requirement.

Black Cohosh	1:2	15 mL
Ginger	1:2	15 mL
Dong Quai	1:2	35 mL
Wild Yam	1:2	35 mL
		100 mL

Dose: 5 mL with water 2 times a day. Symptomatic treatment should also be used as above but taken just prior to menstruation
Chaste Tree 1:2 (2 mL with water on rising) so long as PMS or congestive symptoms are also present

EXAMPLE TABLET/SINGLE LIQUID PROTOCOL

Core Treatment

Smooth Muscle Relaxant (4 to 8 tablets per day) started a few days before painful menstruation is anticipated and discontinued when the painful period has abated

Additional Treatments (as required)

- Chaste Tree (2 tablets on rising throughout the cycle) if congestive or PMS symptoms are also present.
- Dong Quai (2 tablets per day throughout the cycle) if the pain is severe and debilitating.
- Smooth Muscle Relaxant (2 to 3 tablets per day throughout the cycle) if the pain is severe and debilitating.
- Herbal Antioxidant (2 tablets per day as required) for diarrhoea associated with menstruation.
- Liver Detox Assist (2 to 3 tablets per day throughout the cycle) to support hormonal balance by improving hepatic clearance of hormones.

Backup Treatments

If none of the above protocols afford sufficient relief, try one or more of the options below (in addition to the Core Treatment)

- High Potency Willow Bark (4 tablets per day; 2 plus 2) taken on the same days as Smooth Muscle Relaxant for additional analgesic activity.

- Menopause Support (3 tablets per day throughout the cycle) for uterotonic and hormone-balancing effects.
- Paeonia 1:2 (4 mL per day throughout the cycle) or High Potency Tribulus Leaf (2 tablets per day) to restore hormonal balance.

ECZEMA

See Dermatitis

FATIGUE

EXAMPLE LIQUID FORMULATIONS

Licorice	1:1	15 mL
Skullcap	1:2	25 mL
Korean Ginseng	1:2	15 mL
St John's Wort	1:2	20 mL
Withania	1:1	25 mL
		100 mL

Dose: 8 mL with water twice a day

ALTERNATIVE EXAMPLE LIQUID FORMULATION

Siberian Ginseng	1:2	30 mL
Rhodiola	2:1	40 mL
Codonopsis	1:2	30 mL
		100 mL

Dose: 8 mL with water twice a day

Core Treatment

Stress Control (3 to 4 tablets per day)

AND

Stress Adapt (3 to 4 tablets per day)

Additional Treatments (as required)

- Nervous System Tonic (3 to 4 tablets per day) if emotional stress and a depleted nervous system are present.

- Long Term Immune Support (3 to 4 tablets per day), switching to Short Term Immune Support (6 to 8 tablets per day) during acute infections, if recurrent infections are a feature.
- Licorice 1:1 (3 mL per day) if adrenal support is required, especially if the patient has low blood pressure. If Stress Control is already being taken be cautious of raising blood pressure excessively.

FIBROMYALGIA

EXAMPLE LIQUID FORMULATION

Celery Seed	1:2	30 mL
St John's Wort	1:2	20 mL
Valerian	1:2	20 mL
Withania	1:1	25 mL
Feverfew	1:5	10 mL
		105 mL

Dose: 5 mL with water 3 times a day or 8 mL twice a day

EXAMPLE TABLET/SINGLE LIQUID PROTOCOL

Core Treatment

Autoimmune Formula (3 to 4 tablets per day)

AND

Stress Control (4 tablets per day) (alternatively Stress Adapt at 3 tablets per day)

AND

St John's Wort (3 tablets per day)

Additional Treatments (as required)

- Sleep/Anxiety Support (3 tablets about one hour before bed) for associated sleep onset insomnia. Consider also Chaste Tree (2 tablets per day) for sleep maintenance insomnia.
- High Potency Willow Bark (3 to 4 tablets per day) or Boswellia Combination (3 to 4 tablets per day) for painful muscles and joints.

- Echinacea Formula (2 tablets per day) to balance immune function.
- Hawthorn for the autonomic imbalance and circulatory abnormalities (2 tablets per day) and Herbal Thyroid Support (3 tablets per day for the large tablets or 6 per day for the small tablets) if thyroid function is compromised.
- Ginkgo (3 tablets or 3 mL of 2:1 liquid with water per day) to boost cerebral and peripheral blood flow.

FOOD ALLERGIES/SENSITIVITIES

EXAMPLE LIQUID FORMULATION

Echinacea Root blend	1:2	30 mL
Gentiana	1:2	5 mL
Schisandra	1:2	20 mL
Chamomile	1:2	20 mL
Globe Artichoke	1:2	25 mL
		100 mL

Dose: 5 mL with water 3 times a day before meals or 8 mL twice a day

EXAMPLE TABLET/SINGLE LIQUID PROTOCOL

Core Treatment

Upper Digestive Formula (1 tablet 3 times a day before meals, sucked 30 to 60 seconds before swallowing)
AND
Liver/Biliary Tonic (3 to 4 tablets per day)

Additional Treatments (as required)

- Liver Protection Formula (3 tablets per day) especially if there is evidence or history of liver damage or poor liver function.
- Liver Detox Assist (3 to 4 tablets per day) if chemical sensitivity is suspected as part of the food intolerance.
- Allergy Support (3 tablets per day) if classical food allergy is present or there is a strong history of atopy (urticaria, eczema etc).

- Echinacea Formula (2 tablets per day) or Short Term Immune Support (3 tablets per day) if immunity is particularly poor.
- Bowel flora dysbiosis protocol for gut dysbiosis if it is suspected to play a role.

GASTRO-OESOPHAGEAL REFLUX

EXAMPLE LIQUID FORMULATION

Passionflower	1:2	20 mL
Chamomile	1:2	25 mL
Meadowsweet	1:2	25 mL
Licorice	1:1	15 mL
Yarrow	1:2	15 mL
		100 mL

Dose: 5 mL with water 3 times a day after meals. An extra dose can be taken before retiring in the evening. Works best if taken in conjunction with Slippery Elm capsules or powder (also after meals)

EXAMPLE TABLET/SINGLE LIQUID PROTOCOL

Core Treatment

Gastric Mucosal Support (1 to 2 tablets with water after meals and before bed)

Additional Treatments (as required)

- Marshmallow 1:5 glycetract (4 mL with water) or Slippery Elm (3 capsules per time) after meals and before bed to provide additional mucoprotective activity.
- Smooth Muscle Relaxant (3 tablets per day) to restore balance to smooth muscle function.
- Upper Digestive Formula (1 tablet before meals sucked for 30 seconds) to improve sphincter tone and to address any associated dyspepsia.
- Sleep/Anxiety Support (3 tablets per day) to address any associated stress-related anxiety.
- Herbal Antioxidant (2 tablets per day) or Ginkgo (3 tablets per day) for antioxidant activity and favourable effects on microcirculation.

HAYFEVER

EXAMPLE LIQUID FORMULATION

Echinacea Root blend	1:2	35 mL
Eyebright	1:2	20 mL
Golden Seal	1:3	20 mL
Baical Skullcap	1:2	30 mL
		105 mL

Dose: 5 mL with water 3 times a day before meals or 8 mL twice a day

EXAMPLE TABLET/SINGLE LIQUID PROTOCOL

Core Treatment

Upper Respiratory Tract Support (4 tablets per day)
AND
Allergy Support (3 to 4 tablets per day, taken at different times of day to the Upper Respiratory Tract Support)

Additional Treatments (as required)

- Additional Golden Seal (2 tablets per day) if there is excessive mucus discharge.
- Sleep/Anxiety Support (3 tablets per day) or Nervous System Tonic (3 tablets per day) if the allergy is particularly exacerbated by stress.

HERPES SIMPLEX AND SHINGLES

EXAMPLE LIQUID FORMULATION

For acute outbreaks the following formula has helped several patients in conjunction with topical application of Calendula 1:2 extract

Echinacea Root blend	1:2	70 mL
St John's Wort (high in hypericin)	1:2	30 mL
		100 mL

Dose: 5 mL with water 4 to 5 times a day until the lesions heal

EXAMPLE TABLET/SINGLE LIQUID PROTOCOL

Core Treatment

For prevention:
Echinacea Formula (2 to 3 tablets per day)
AND
St John's Wort (3 tablets per day)
For acute outbreaks:
Double the above doses of both formulations

Additional Treatments (as required)

- Stress Control (3 to 4 tablets per day) or Long Term Immune Support (3 to 4 tablets per day) for debilitated patients suffering recurrent outbreaks.
- Topical treatment of lesions with Lemon Balm 1:2, or Licorice 1:1 and/or Calendula 1:2 incorporated into a suitable base. Topical treatment of painful dermatomes with a Cayenne cream for post-herpetic neuralgia.

HYPERTHYROIDISM

EXAMPLE LIQUID FORMULATION

Bugleweed	1:2	20 mL
Motherwort	1:2	20 mL
Echinacea Root blend	1:2	20 mL
Bupleurum	1:2	25 mL
St John's Wort (high in hypericin)	1:2	20 mL
		105 mL

Dose: 5 to 8 mL with water 3 times a day or 8 mL twice a day

EXAMPLE TABLET/SINGLE LIQUID PROTOCOL

Core Treatment

Bugleweed 1:2 (4 mL with water per day)
AND
Echinacea Formula (2 to 3 tablets per day)

AND
Autoimmune Formula (3 or 4 tablets per day)

Additional Treatments (as required)

- St John's Wort (3 to 4 tablets per day) if a viral aetiology is suspected.
- Motherwort 1:2 (3 to 4 mL with water per day) if cardiac symptoms such as tachycardia and palpitations are present.
- Bowel flora dysbiosis protocol.

HYPOTHYROIDISM

EXAMPLE LIQUID FORMULATION

Bladderwrack	1:1	40 mL
Coleus	1:1	35 mL
Withania	1:1	25 mL
		100 mL

Dose: 5 mL with water 3 times a day or 8 mL twice a day

EXAMPLE TABLET/SINGLE LIQUID PROTOCOL

Core Treatment

Herbal Thyroid Support (3 to 4 tablets per day for the large tablets or 6 to 9 tablets per day for the small tablets)

Additional Treatments (as required)

- Echinacea Formula (2 to 3 tablets per day) for immune modulation.
- St John's Wort (3 to 4 tablets per day) for antiviral activity against enveloped viruses.
- Autoimmune Formula (3 to 4 tablets per day) for anti-inflammatory activity.
- Bowel flora dysbiosis protocol.

Backup Treatment

Coleus Forskohlii (2 to 3 tablets per day) as appropriate in addition to the above

IMPOTENCE

EXAMPLE LIQUID FORMULATION

Ginkgo	2:1	20 mL
Korean Ginseng	1:2	15 mL
Saw Palmetto	1:2	25 mL
Damiana	1:2	20 mL
Rhodiola	2:1	20 mL
		100 mL

Dose: 5 mL with water 3 times a day or 8 mL twice a day

EXAMPLE TABLET/SINGLE LIQUID PROTOCOL

Core Treatment

High Potency Tribulus Leaf (3 to 4 tablets per day)

Additional Treatments (as required)

- If the patient has performance anxiety include Sleep/Anxiety Support (3 to 4 tablets per day).
- If the patient is devitalised and low in mood consider as appropriate Nervous System Tonic (3 to 4 tablets per day) or Stress Control (3 to 4 tablets per day) or Rhodiola 2:1 (4 mL with water once a day).
- If a basically healthy patient suffers impotence as a result of heavy stress add Stress Adapt (3 tablets per day).
- If adrenal function is low add Rehmannia 1:2 (4 mL with water once a day).
- If the patient has poor circulation recommend Ginkgo (3 to 4 tablets per day).

Backup Treatment

Korean Ginseng 1:2 (3 mL with water per day)
AND
Saw Palmetto 1:2 (4 mL with water per day)

INFERTILITY, FEMALE

EXAMPLE LIQUID FORMULATIONS

Paeonia	1:2	25 mL
Wild Yam	1:2	30 mL
Chaste Tree	1:2	15 mL
Dong Quai	1:2	30 mL
		100 mL

Dose: 5 mL with water 3 times a day or 8 mL twice a day

ALTERNATIVE LIQUID FORMULATION

Paeonia	1:2	30 mL
Shatavari	1:2	35 mL
Chaste Tree	1:2	15 mL
Licorice	1:1	20 mL
		100 mL

Dose: 5 mL 3 to 4 times a day or 8 mL 2 to 3 times a day

EXAMPLE TABLET/SINGLE LIQUID PROTOCOL

Core Treatment

The following treatment will help to establish or maintain ovulation and normal reproductive function:

Chaste Tree (2 tablets on rising each day)

AND

High Potency Tribulus Leaf (3 tablets per day on days 5 to 14 inclusive of the menstrual cycle: the first day of menstruation is day 1)

Additional Treatments (as required)

- Black Cohosh 1:2 (2 mL with water once a day) to improve ovarian function.
- Dong Quai (2 tablets per day) as a female tonic.
- Paeonia 1:2 (4 mL with water once a day) to normalise folliculogenesis.

- Stress Adapt (3 tablets per day) to treat any adverse effects of stress, especially in idiopathic infertility.
- Smooth Muscle Relaxant (3 tablets per day) for suspected oviductal spasm in idiopathic fertility.
- Nervous System Tonic (3 tablets per day) for the patient suffering idiopathic infertility who is low in nervous energy.
- Anxiety Support or Sleep/Anxiety Support (3 tablets per day) for the anxious patient with idiopathic infertility.
- Stress Control (3 tablets per day) for the exhausted or depleted patient with idiopathic infertility.
- Rehmannia 1:2 or Licorice 1:1 (high in glycyrrhizin) (4 mL with water per day of either) if there are indications of excessive stress-related symptoms and adrenal insufficiency.

INFERTILITY, MALE

EXAMPLE LIQUID FORMULATION

Korean Ginseng	1:2	25 mL
Saw Palmetto	1:2	25 mL
Ginkgo	2:1	20 mL
Withania	1:1	30 mL
		100 mL

Dose: 5 mL with water 3 times a day or 8 mL twice a day

EXAMPLE TABLET/SINGLE LIQUID PROTOCOL

Core Treatment

High Potency Tribulus Leaf (3 to 4 tablets per day)

Additional Treatments (as required)

- Prostate Support (3 to 4 capsules per day) if a history of prostatitis is thought to be a contributory factor.
- Herbal Antioxidant (2 tablets per day) for antioxidant effects and improving microcirculation.
- Stress Control (3 to 4 tablets per day) if the patient is stressed and debilitated.

Backup Treatment

Korean Ginseng 1:2 (3 mL with water once a day)
AND
Saw Palmetto 1:2 (4 mL with water once a day)

INSOMNIA

EXAMPLE LIQUID FORMULATIONS

Sleep Onset Insomnia

Valerian	1:2	25 mL
Passionflower	1:2	20 mL
Zizyphus	1:2	25 mL
Withania	1:1	30 mL
		100 mL

Dose: 5 mL with water 3 times a day. Take the last dose one hour before bed

Sleep Maintenance or Sleep Offset Insomnia

Valerian	1:2	25 mL
St John's Wort	1:2	30 mL
Chaste Tree	1:2	20 mL
Skullcap	1:2	25 mL
		100 mL

Dose: 5 mL with water 3 times a day. Take the last dose one hour before bed

EXAMPLE TABLET/SINGLE LIQUID PROTOCOL

Core Treatment

Sleep/Anxiety Support (4 to 6 tablets per day. 2 or 3 tablets can be taken throughout the day, with 2 or 3 tablets recommended about one hour before retiring). Best results will come with continuous use for at least 2 weeks. Can be used for both sleep onset and sleep maintenance insomnia
OR
Alternatively try Anxiety Support (3 to 4 tablets per day)

Additional Treatments (depending on the type of insomnia)

- Nervous System Tonic (3 to 4 tablets during the day) for sleep maintenance (or sleep offset insomnia) or alternatively try Chaste Tree (3 tablets throughout the day). In those cases the Sleep/Anxiety Support or Anxiety Support tablets could only be taken at night at a dose of 2 to 3 tablets one hour before bed.
- If sleep maintenance insomnia is thought to be caused by nocturnal hypoglycaemia then Rehmannia 1:2 (4 mL with water) or Licorice 1:1 (3 mL with water) should be taken in the evening.
- For non-restorative sleep Stress Control (3 to 4 tablets per day) or Withania 1:1 (5 mL with water once a day) can be recommended during the day. Alternatively try Rhodiola 2:1 (4 mL with water) just before bed.
- High Potency Willow Bark for musculoskeletal pain (2 to 4 tablets per day) or Smooth Muscle Relaxant for cramping pain in smooth muscle (3 to 4 tablets per day) can be added if pain interferes with sleep.
- For restless legs syndrome Vein Formula (2 to 3 tablets per day).

IRRITABLE BOWEL SYNDROME

EXAMPLE LIQUID FORMULATION

Ginger	1:2	10 mL
Meadowsweet	1:2	20 mL
Fringe Tree	1:2	15 mL
St Mary's Thistle	1:1	20 mL
Chamomile	1:2	20 mL
Cramp Bark	1:2	20 mL
		105 mL

Dose: 5 mL with water 3 times a day or 8 mL twice a day
Slippery Elm powder or capsules combine well with this formulation

EXAMPLE TABLET/SINGLE LIQUID PROTOCOL

Core Treatment

Nervous System Tonic (3 to 4 tablets per day)

AND

Smooth Muscle Relaxant (3 tablets per day)

AND

Chamomile 1:2 (4 mL with water per day)

Additional Treatments (as required)

- Liver/Biliary Tonic (3 to 4 tablets per day) to improve bile flow and treat any associated constipation.
- Liver Protection Formula (2 to 3 tablets per day) if the IBS is associated with liver damage or a recent history of hepatitis.
- Sleep/Anxiety Support (3 to 4 tablets per day) instead of the Nervous System Tonic if the patient suffers from anxiety.
- Boswellia Combination (3 tablets per day) and Allergy Support (3 tablets per day) instead of the Nervous System Tonic if inflammation and allergy are thought to be the primary cause.
- Chaste Tree (2 tablets per day on rising) if symptoms are worse premenstrually.

Backup Treatment

Follow the protocol for Bowel flora dysbiosis outlined in this book in addition to the Core Treatment above

LIVER DIGESTIVE FUNCTION, TO IMPROVE

EXAMPLE LIQUID FORMULATION

St Mary's Thistle	1:1	30 mL
Globe Artichoke	1:2	25 mL
Schisandra	1:2	25 mL
Dandelion Root	1:2	20 mL
		100 mL

Dose: 5 mL with water 3 times a day before meals or 8 mL twice a day

EXAMPLE TABLET/SINGLE LIQUID PROTOCOL

Core Treatment

Liver/Biliary Tonic (3 to 4 tablets per day)

Additional Treatment (as required)

- Liver Protection Formula (2 to 3 tablets per day) if there is a history of liver damage.

LIVER PHASE I/II DETOXIFICATION, TO IMPROVE

EXAMPLE LIQUID FORMULATION

Schisandra	1:2	25 mL
St Mary's Thistle	1:2	25 mL
Rosemary	1:2	30 mL
Turmeric	1:1	25 mL
		105 mL

Dose: 5 mL with water 3 times a day or 8 mL twice per day

EXAMPLE TABLET/SINGLE LIQUID PROTOCOL

Core Treatment

Liver Detox Assist (3 to 4 tablets per day)

AND

Herbal Antioxidant (2 tablets per day)

Additional Treatments (as required)

- Liver Protection Formula (2 to 3 tablets per day) if there is history or evidence of liver damage.
- High Allicin Releasing Garlic (1 to 2 tablets per day) for further support for Phase II processes.

MENOPAUSE

EXAMPLE LIQUID FORMULATION

Wild Yam	1:2	20 mL
Shatavari	1:2	20 mL
Sage	1:2	20 mL
St John's Wort	1:2	25 mL
Chaste Tree	1:2	15 mL
		100 mL

Dose: 5 mL with water 3 times a day or 8 mL twice a day

EXAMPLE TABLET/SINGLE LIQUID PROTOCOL

Core Treatment
Menopause Support (3 to 6 tablets per day)

Additional Treatments (as required)
- Chaste Tree (2 tablets per day) if PMS-like symptoms are evident.
- Extra Sage as a 1:2 liquid (4 mL with water per day) if heat symptoms, sweating and hot flushes are not relieved by the Menopause Support.
- Rehmannia 1:2 or Licorice 1:1 (high in glycyrrhizin) (4 mL with water per day of either) if there are indications of excessive stress-related symptoms and adrenal insufficiency.
- Anxiety Support (2 to 3 tablets per day) if anxiety symptoms predominate.
- Extra St John's Wort (2 to 3 tablets per day) if symptoms of depression predominate.

Backup Treatments
If the above Protocols do not afford sufficient relief from symptoms, try adding (to the Core Treatment) one or more of the options below:
- Black Cohosh 1:2 (2 mL with water per day).
- High Potency Tribulus Leaf (3 tablets per day).
- Hawthorn (2 to 3 tablets per day).

- Motherwort 1:2 (4 mL with water per day).
- Ladies Mantle 1:2 (5 mL with water per day).

METABOLIC SYNDROME X

EXAMPLE LIQUID FORMULATION

Licorice	1:1	30 mL
Coleus	1:1	25 mL
Korean Ginseng	1:2	15 mL
Globe Artichoke	1:2	30 mL
		100 mL

Dose: 8 mL with water twice a day

This formulation will provide support for fat loss, stress, glycaemic control and the cardiovascular, pro-inflammatory and pro-oxidant metabolic disturbances

Substitute Hawthorn Leaves 1:2 for Licorice for hyptertension

EXAMPLE TABLET/SINGLE LIQUID PROTOCOL

Weight Loss/Fat Loss
- Coleus Forskohlii (1 tablet before each meal).
- A low glycaemic index protein powder for meal replacement (at least one meal per day) 25 g serve.
- Licorice 1:1 (5 mL with water per day).

Insulin Resistance/Enhanced Glycaemic Control (select as required)
- Liver Protection Formula (1 tablet before each meal).
- Glucose Metabolism Support (1 tablet before each meal).
- Korean Ginseng 1:2 (2 mL with water twice a day before meals).
- Fenugreek 1:2 (4 mL with water twice a day before meals).
- Herbal Antioxidant (1 tablet twice a day before meals).

Cardiovascular Metabolic Disturbances (select as required)
- High Allicin Releasing Garlic (2 tablets per day) for effects of hypertension, elevated LDL-cholesterol and triglycerides and other favourable cardiovascular effects (eg phyto-HDL).

- Hawthorn (3 tablets per day) for hypertension.
- Coleus Forskohlii (dosage as above) for hypertension.

Pro-oxidant/Pro-inflammatory Metabolic Disturbances (select as required)
- Liver Protection Formula (1 tablet before each meal) for antioxidant activity and to reduce Fe stores.
- Herbal Antioxidant (1 tablet twice a day before meals) for antioxidant and anti-inflammatory activity.

Stress Management (select as required)
- Stress Control (3 to 4 tablets per day).
- Korean Ginseng 1:2 (2 to 3 mL with water per day).

OSTEOARTHRITIS

EXAMPLE LIQUID FORMULATIONS

Celery Seed	1:2	30 mL
Devil's Claw	1:2	45 mL
Ginger	1:2	10 mL
Prickly Ash	1:2	20 mL
		105 mL

Dose: 5 mL with water 3 times a day or 8 mL twice a day

Celery Seed	1:2	40 mL
Dandelion Leaf	1:1	30 mL
Ginger	1:2	10 mL
Nettle Leaf	1:2	25 mL
		105 mL

Dose: 5 mL with water 3 times a day or 8 mL twice a day

EXAMPLE TABLET/SINGLE LIQUID PROTOCOL

Core Treatment
Boswellia Combination (4 to 6 tablets per day taken with meals)

Additional Treatments (as required)
- High Potency Willow Bark (2 to 4 tablets per day) if pain is a substantial feature.
- Extra Celery Seed 1:2 (5 mL with water per day) or Nettle Leaf 1:2 (5 mL with water per day) for additional anti-inflammatory and disease-modifying activities.
- Herbs for circulation, especially High Allicin Releasing Garlic (1 to 2 tablets per day) and Ginkgo (3 tablets per day) if there are general symptoms of circulatory deficiency.
- St John's Wort (3 to 4 tablets per day) if nerve entrapment is present.
- Herbal Antioxidant (2 tablets per day) for additional antioxidant effects.
- Gotu Kola 1:1 (4 mL with water 1 to 2 times a day) for chondrocyte integrity.
- Skin/Elimination Support (3 tablets per day) as a long-term depurative treatment.

PMS

EXAMPLE LIQUID FORMULATION

Chaste Tree	1:2	10 mL
St John's Wort	1:2	20 mL
Schisandra	1:2	25 mL
Withania	1:1	25 mL
Skullcap	1:2	30 mL
		110 mL

Dose: 8 mL with water twice a day
If fluid retention is present as a predominating symptom, Dandelion Leaf 1:1 at 8 mL once a day could be added in the second half of the cycle

EXAMPLE TABLET/SINGLE LIQUID PROTOCOL

Core Treatment

Chaste tree (2 tablets per day)

AND

Nervous System Tonic (3 to 4 tablets per day)

Additional Treatments (as required)

- Liver Detox Assist (3 to 4 tablets per day) if signs of liver sluggishness are present.
- Anxiety Support or Sleep/Anxiety Support (3 tablets of either per day) if symptoms of insomnia or anxiety predominate. Perhaps use instead of Nervous System Tonic.
- Stress Adapt (3 tablets per day) or Stress Control (3 to 4 tablets per day) if the patient is showing signs of being under stress.
- Evening Primrose Oil (3 capsules per day) or Ginkgo (3 tablets per day) if mastalgia predominates.
- Dandelion Leaf 1:1 (4 to 8 mL with water per day only during the PMS phase) if fluid retention is a problem.
- Vein Formula (2 tablets per day) if congestive dysmenorrhoea symptoms (pain and congestion around menstruation which lasts for several days) are associated with the PMS.
- Additional St John's Wort (2 tablets per day) if depression is a dominating feature of the PMS.
- Rehmannia 1:2 or Licorice 1:1 (high in glycyrrhizin) (4 mL with water per day of either) if there are indications of excessive stress-related symptoms and adrenal insufficiency/depletion.

Backup Treatments

If none of the above protocols afford sufficient relief of the PMS symptoms try one or more of the options below (either instead of or in addition to the Core Treatment):

- Black Cohosh 1:2 (2 mL with water per day).
- Evening Primrose Oil (3 capsules per day).
- Menopause Support (3 to 4 tablets per day).

- Paeonia 1:2 (4 mL with water per day).
- Dong Quai (2 to 3 tablets per day).

PROSTATITIS, CHRONIC

EXAMPLE LIQUID FORMULATION

Echinacea Root blend	1:2	25 mL
Saw Palmetto	1:2	20 mL
Licorice	1:1	15 mL
Buchu	1:2	20 mL
Crataeva	1:2	30 mL
		110 mL

Dose: 5 mL with water 3 times a day or 8 mL twice a day

EXAMPLE TABLET/SINGLE LIQUID PROTOCOL

Core Treatment

Prostate Support (2 to 3 capsules per day)

AND

Echinacea Formula (2 to 3 tablets per day)

Additional Treatments (as required)

- Urinary Tract Support (4 tablets per day) to control a bacterial presence.
- If the patient has chronic poor immunity Long Term Immune Support (3 to 4 tablets per day) instead of the Echinacea.
- Additional support for the prostate tissue with Nettle Root 1:2 (4 mL with water per day) and/or Golden Seal (2 tablets per day).
- Mushroom Immune Formula (3 to 4 tablets per day) for secretory IgA deficiency.
- Herbal Antioxidant (2 tablets per day) to reduce oxidative stress.

Backup Treatments

If the patient's case does not respond to the above protocol then treat as prostatodynia. Consider selecting from the following:

- Prostate Support (3 to 4 capsules per day) and/or Nettle Root 1:2 (4 mL with water per day) to support the prostate gland.
- Smooth Muscle Relaxant (3 to 4 tablets per day) for pain and spasm in the prostate.
- Stress Control (3 to 4 tablets per day) or Nervous System Tonic (3 to 4 tablets per day) to boost energy and resistance to stress.
- Autoimmune Support (3 to 4 tablets per day) to help control any associated inflammation.

REACTIVE HYPOGLYCAEMIA

See Dysglycaemia

RHEUMATOID ARTHRITIS

EXAMPLE LIQUID FORMULATION

Echinacea Root blend	1:2	30 mL
St John's Wort (high in hypericin)	1:2	20 mL
Bupleurum	1:2	20 mL
Cat's Claw	1:2	25 mL
Ginger	1:2	10 mL
		105 mL

Dose: 5 mL with water 3 times a day or 8 mL twice a day

EXAMPLE TABLET/SINGLE LIQUID PROTOCOL

Core Treatment

Cat's Claw Immune Formula (4 tablets per day)

AND

Boswellia Combination (3 to 4 tablets per day)

AND

Bowel flora dysbiosis protocol

Additional Treatments (as required)

- St John's Wort (3 to 4 tablets per day) for antiviral activity against enveloped viruses.

- Autoimmune Formula (3 to 4 tablets per day) for additional anti-inflammatory activity.
- Urinary Tract Support (3 to 6 tablets per day) for Proteus in the urine.

SINUSITIS, CHRONIC

EXAMPLE LIQUID FORMULATION

Echinacea Root blend	1:2	40 mL
Eyebright	1:2	30 mL
Golden Seal	1:3	25 mL
Poke Root	1:5	5 mL
		100 mL

Dose: 5 mL with water 3 times a day or 8 mL twice a day

EXAMPLE TABLET/SINGLE LIQUID PROTOCOL

Core Treatment

Upper Respiratory Tract Support (4 tablets per day)

AND

Short Term Immune Support (4 tablets per day)

Additional Treatments (as required)

- Golden Seal (2 to 4 tablets per day) if mucus discharge is green/yellow and excessive.
- High Allicin Releasing Garlic (2 tablets per day) if mucus is thick and does not easily drain from the sinuses.
- Long Term Immune Support (3 to 4 tablets per day) instead of the Short Term Immune Support if there is weakened immunity or night sweats.
- Allergy Support (3 to 4 tablets per day) if there is a strong history and current manifestations of allergy.

Backup Treatment

Cat's Claw Immune Formula (4 tablets per day) as an antifungal treatment

AND

Upper Respiratory Tract Support (4 tablets per day)

AND
Poke Root 1:5 (0.5 mL per day with water – CAUTION: Do not exceed recommended dose)

ULCERATIVE COLITIS

EXAMPLE LIQUID FORMULATION

Echinacea Root blend	1:2	30 mL
Chamomile	1:2	20 mL
St John's Wort	1:2	25 mL
Bupleurum	1:2	20 mL
Licorice	1:1	15 mL
		110 mL

Dose: 5 mL with water 3 times a day or 8 mL twice a day
For best results combine with Boswellia Combination (3 to 4 tablets per day) and the Bowel flora dysbiosis protocol on an ongoing basis

EXAMPLE TABLET/SINGLE LIQUID PROTOCOL

Core Treatment
Echinacea Formula (2 to 3 tablets per day)
AND
Boswellia Combination (3 to 4 tablets per day)
AND
The Bowel flora dysbiosis protocol on a long-term basis

Additional Treatments (as required)
- Autoimmune Formula (3 to 4 tablets per day) to allay immune-mediated inflammation.
- St John's Wort (3 to 4 tablets per day) if a viral association is suspected.
- Golden Seal (3 to 4 tablets per day) as an alternative to the Bowel flora dysbiosis protocol.

VARICOSE VEINS AND HAEMORRHOIDS

EXAMPLE LIQUID FORMULATION

Horsechestnut	1:2	30 mL
Ginkgo	2:1	20 mL
Butcher's Broom	1:2	20 mL
Gotu Kola	1:1	30 mL
		100 mL

Dose: 5 mL with water 2 to 3 times a day or 8 mL twice a day

CREAM

Cream base		40 g
Witch Hazel	1:2	7 mL
Horsechestnut	1:2	7 mL

Blend together and place in a sterile jar with a suitable label.
Apply 2 to 3 times a day

EXAMPLE TABLET/SINGLE LIQUID PROTOCOL

Core Treatment
Vein Formula (2 to 3 tablets per day)

Additional Treatments (as required)
- Herbal Antioxidant (2 tablets per day) and/or Bilberry (3 to 4 tablets per day) to improve microcirculation.
- Echinacea Formula (3 tablets per day) if varicose ulcers are present.

Backup Treatment
- Gotu Kola 1:1 (4 mL with water twice a day)

WEIGHT LOSS, TO ASSIST

See also Metabolic syndrome X

EXAMPLE LIQUID FORMULATION

Coleus	1:1	35 mL
Gymnema	1:1	35 mL
Bladderwrack	1:1	35 mL
		105 mL

Dose: 5 mL with water 3 times a day or 8 mL twice a day

Note: This formulation may need to be flavoured as the taste will be extremely unpleasant

EXAMPLE TABLET/SINGLE LIQUID PROTOCOL

Core Treatment

Coleus Forskohlii (2 to 3 tablets per day before meals)

AND

Glucose Metabolism Support (2 to 3 tablets per day before meals)

Additional Treatments (as required)

- Herbal Thyroid Support (3 to 4 tablets per day for the large tablets or 6 to 9 tablets per day for the small tablets) for poor thyroid activity or subclinical hypothyroidism.
- Licorice 1:1 (5 mL with water per day for fat loss).

WORMS, INTESTINAL

EXAMPLE LIQUID FORMULATION

Echinacea Root blend	1:2	30 mL
Wormwood	1:5	15 mL
Black Walnut Hulls	1:10	20 mL
Cranesbill Root	1:2	20 mL
Thyme	1:2	25 mL
		110 mL

Dose: 5 mL with water 4 to 6 times a day for 10 days. After a 10-day break, repeat treatment for 10 days. The second treatment is to kill any larvae which may have hatched after treatment, since herbal anthelmintics are not very effective at killing eggs

Note: These are adult doses. For children's doses use the calculation provided in the How to Use section

EXAMPLE TABLET/SINGLE LIQUID PROTOCOL

Note: The doses for products given below represent adult doses. For children's doses use the calculation provided in the How to Use section

Core Treatment

Short Term Immune Support (4 to 6 tablets per day as a continuous treatment)

AND

Wormwood Combination (4 to 6 tablets per day for 10 days. After a 10-day break, repeat treatment for 10 days)

Additional Treatments (as required)

- High Allicin Releasing Garlic (3 tablets per day on the same days as the Wormwood Combination) for stubborn parasites.
- Upper Digestive Formula (1 tablet before each meal sucked for 30 to 60 seconds) if a low gastric acid barrier and poor digestion are thought to contribute to reinfestation.
- Herbal Antioxidant (2 tablets per day) on the same days as the Wormwood Combination but at different times to provide synergistic worm-killing activity.
- Herbal Bowel Support (2 to 6 tablets before bed twice a week) during treatment with the Wormwood Combination to assist the expulsion of worms. The dose should be sufficient to create a very loose stool.

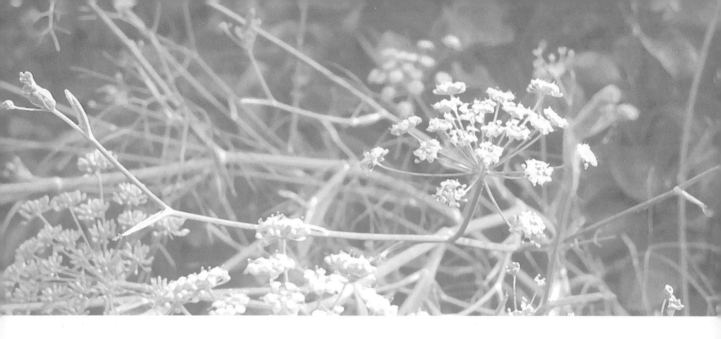

Contraindications and Cautions

General, including Pregnancy

ACUTE INFECTIONS

Caution

- Astragalus
- Dong Quai
- Korean Ginseng
- Siberian Ginseng

BRADYCARDIA

Contraindicated

- Jamaica Dogwood

CARDIAC INSUFFICIENCY

Contraindicated

- Jamaica Dogwood
- Licorice (in high doses)

CHILDREN

Contraindicated

- Bearberry (if under 12)

Caution

- Aloes Resin
- Cascara
- Garlic
- Pasque Flower
- Rhubarb Root
- Senna Pods

CHOLESTASIS

Caution

- Tribulus

DAMAGED SKIN

Contraindicated topically

- Arnica
- Horsechestnut
- Comfrey
- Horseradish
- Poke Root

Caution topically

- Cayenne

DEPRESSION

Contraindicated

- Hops

DIARRHOEA

Contraindicated

- Cascara
- Senna Pods

Caution

- Zizyphus

EPILEPSY

Caution

- Thuja

GALLSTONES

Caution

- Ginger

GASTRO-OESOPHAGEAL REFLUX

Contraindicated

- Peppermint

Caution

- Angelica Root
- Aniseed
- Bacopa
- Beth Root
- Bupleurum
- Butcher's Broom
- Cayenne
- Cinnamon
- Cloves
- Dill
- False Unicorn
- Fennel
- Fenugreek
- Gentian
- Ginger
- Gymnema
- Horsechestnut
- Polygala
- Sarsaparilla
- Shatavari
- Tribulus
- Wild Yam
- Wormwood

GASTROINTESTINAL INFLAMMATION

Contraindicated

- Poke Root

Caution

- Aloes Resin
- Cascara
- Rhubarb Root
- Senna Pods

GLUCOSE-6 DEHYDROGENESE DEFICIENCY

Contraindicated

- Willow Bark

HEAVY MENSTRUATION

Caution

- Dong-Quai

HYPERTENSION

Contraindicated

- Kola Nut
- Licorice (in high doses)

Caution

- Korean Ginseng

HYPERTHYROIDISM

Contraindicated

- Bladderwrack

HYPOKALAEMIA

Contraindicated

Licorice (in high doses)

HYPOTENSION

Contraindicated

Coleus

HYPOTHYROIDISM

Contraindicated

Bugleweed
Horseradish (high doses only)

INSOMNIA

Contraindicated

Kola Nut

INTERNAL USE

Contraindicated

Arnica
Comfrey

INTESTINAL OBSTRUCTION

Contraindicated

Slippery Elm

IRRITABLE BOWEL SYNDROME

Caution

Aloes Resin
Cascara
Rhubarb Root
Senna Pods

KIDNEY DISEASE

Contraindicated

Bearberry
Sheep Sorrel

Caution

Licorice (in high doses)

KIDNEY STONES

Caution

Cranberry (oxalate stones)

LACTATION

Contraindicated

Barberry
Bearberry
Bladderwrack
Blue Cohosh
Golden Seal
Mugwort
Oregon Grape
Pasque Flower
Poke Root
Sage (except to stop milk)
Thuja
Tylophora
Willow Bark
Wormwood

Caution

Aloes Resin
Cascara
Peppermint
Rhubarb Root
Senna Pods
Shepherd's Purse

LIVER DISEASE

Contraindicated

Chaparral
Greater Celandine

Caution

Licorice (in high doses)
Kava (only use aqueous extract)

LYMPHOCYTIC LEUKAEMIA

Contraindicated

Poke Root

OEDEMA

Contraindicated

Licorice (in high doses)

OESTROGEN-SENSITIVE BREAST CANCER

Best Avoided

Alfalfa
Black Cohosh (controversial, may be safe)
Hops

PEPTIC ULCERS

Contraindicated

Coleus
Horseradish
Kola Nut

Caution

Angelica Root
Cayenne
Devil's Claw
Gentian
Ginger
Wormwood

PHOTOSENSITIVITY

Caution

Angelica Root
St John's Wort

PREGNANCY

Contraindicated

Adhatoda (except at birth)
Andrographis (first trimester)
Baical Skullcap (first trimester)
Barberry
Bearberry
Black Cohosh (except to assist with birth)
Bladderwrack
Blue Cohosh (except to assist with birth)
Cat's Claw
Corydalis
Dan Shen
Dong-Quai (first trimester)

Contraindicated (cont.)

- Golden Seal
- Horseradish (high doses only)
- Hyssop
- Jamaica Dogwood
- Juniper
- Mugwort
- Myrrh
- Oregon Grape
- Pasque Flower
- Pau D'Arco
- Poke Root
- Qing Hao
- Sage
- Schisandra (except at birth)
- Thuja
- Tienchi Ginseng
- Tylophora
- Wormwood

Caution

- Aloes Resin
- Cascara
- Cinnamon
- Ginger
- Motherwort
- Raspberry Leaf (best to use in 2nd and 3rd trimester)
- Rehmannia
- Rhubarb Root
- Senna Pods
- Shepherd's Purse

SALICYLATE SENSITIVITY

Contraindicated

- Meadowsweet
- Willow Bark

SHORT-TERM USE ONLY

- Aloes resin
- Cascara
- Cranesbill
- Greater Celandine
- Lomatium (long-term use may cause rash)
- Myrrh
- Rhubarb Root (if high doses)
- Sage
- Senna Pods
- Tylophora
- Wild Cherry

SPASMODIC DYSMENORRHOEA

Caution

- Chaste Tree

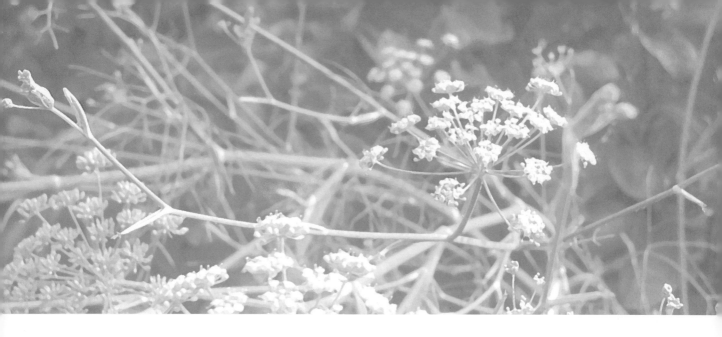

Contraindications and Cautions

Herb/Drug Interactions

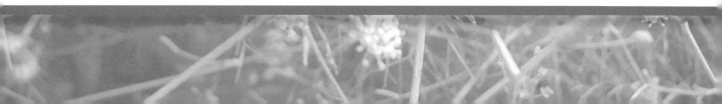

ANTIDIABETIC DRUGS

Caution with

Cinnamon
Goat's Rue

ANTIPLATELET DRUGS

Contraindicated with

Dan Shen

Caution with

Bilberry (high doses)
Coleus
Garlic
Turmeric (high doses)
Willow Bark

CAFFEINE AND CNS STIMULANTS

Caution with

Korean Ginseng
Rhodiola

CONTRACEPTIVE PILL

Contraindicated with

St John's Wort (high hyperforin preparations)

Caution with

Chaste Tree

CYCLOSPORIN

Contraindicated with

St John's Wort (high hyperforin preparations)

DIGOXIN

Contraindicated with

Cascara
Senna Pods
St John's Wort (high hyperforin preparations)

Caution with

Hawthorn
Licorice (in high doses)

DIURETICS

Caution with

Licorice (in high doses)

HIV DRUGS

Contraindicated with

St John's Wort (high hyperforin preparations)

HYPOTENSIVE DRUGS

Caution with

Coleus

IMATINIB

Contraindicated with

St John's Wort (high hyperforin preparations)

IMMUNOSUPPRESSIVE DRUGS

Caution with

Andrographis
Astragalus
Cat's Claw
Echinacea Root
Poke Root

IRINOTECAN

Contraindicated with

St John's Wort (high hyperforin preparations)

LAXATIVES

Caution with

Licorice (in high doses)

MAOI ANTIDEPRESSANTS

Contraindicated with

Korean Ginseng

METHADONE

Contraindicated with

St John's Wort (high hyperforin preparations)

MINERAL SUPPLEMENTS, THIAMINE OR ALKALOIDS

Take away from

Bayberry
Bearberry
Cinnamon
Cranesbill
Grape Seed
Green Tea
Hawthorn
Lime Flowers
Meadowsweet
Pelargonium
Peppermint
Raspberry Leaf
Rhodiola
Rhubarb Root
Rosemary
Vervain
Willow Herb
Witch Hazel

PRESCRIBED DRUGS

Take away from

Marshmallow
Slippery Elm

Caution with

Coleus
St John's Wort (high hyperforin preparations)

PROGESTERONE DRUGS

Caution with

Chaste Tree

SAQUINAVIR

Caution with

Garlic

VERAPAMIL

Contraindicated with

St John's Wort (high hyperforin preparations)

WARFARIN

Contraindicated with

Dan Shen
Korean Ginseng
Pau D'Arco
St John's Wort (high hyperforin preparations)

Caution with

Cranberry
Dong Quai
Garlic
Ginger
Ginkgo (low risk)
Meadowsweet
Saw Palmetto
Turmeric (high doses)
Willow Bark

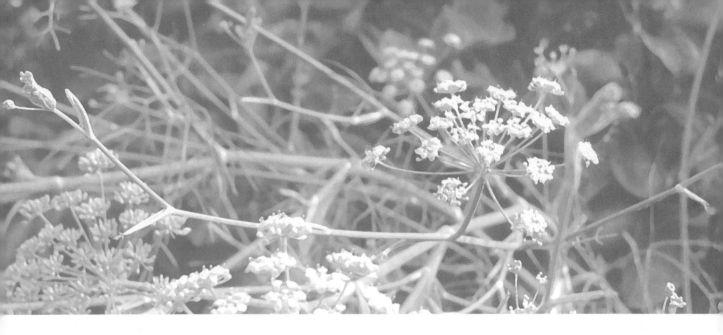

Appendix 1

Glossary of Herbal Actions

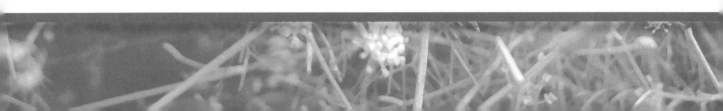

ADAPTOGENIC

A substance that increases the body's resistance or adaptation to physical, environmental, emotional or biological stressors and promotes normal physiological function

ADRENAL TONIC

A substance that improves the tone, histology and function of the adrenal glands (especially the cortex).

ALTERATIVE

See Depurative

ANALGESIC

A substance that relieves pain

ANAPHRODISIAC

A substance that reduces libido (usually in males)

ANODYNE

See Analgesic

ANTACID

A substance that counteracts or neutralises acidity in the gastrointestinal tract

ANTHELMINTIC

A substance that kills or assists in the expulsion of intestinal worms

ANTIALLERGIC

A substance that tones down the allergic response, often by stabilising mast cells

ANTIANDROGENIC

A substance that inhibits or modifies the action of androgens (male sex hormones)

ANTIANAEMIC

A substance that prevents or corrects anaemia (that is a reduction in the number of circulating red blood cells or in the quantity of haemoglobin)

ANTIARRHYTHMIC

A substance that prevents or is effective against arrhythmias (that are any variation from the normal rhythm or rate of the heart beat)

ANTIASTHMATIC

A substance that prevents or relieves asthma attacks

ANTIBACTERIAL

A substance that inhibits the growth of bacteria (bacteriostatic) or destroys bacteria (bactericidal)

ANTICARIOGENIC

A substance that reduces the incidence of dental caries (tooth decay)

ANTICATARRHAL

A substance that reduces the formation of catarrh or phlegm (pathological mucus secretion)

ANTICOAGULANT

A substance that reduces the rate of blood coagulation

ANTICONVULSANT

A substance that tends to prevent or arrest seizures (convulsions)

ANTIDEPRESSANT

A substance that alleviates depression

ANTIDIABETIC

See also Hypoglycaemic

A substance that alleviates diabetes or the effects of diabetes

ANTIDIARRHOEAL

A substance that alleviates diarrhoea

ANTIECCHYMOTIC

A substance that prevents or alleviates bruising

ANTIEMETIC

A substance that reduces nausea and vomiting

ANTIFIBROTIC

A substance that reduces the excessive formulation of fibrous connective tissue, eg in scleroderma

ANTIFUNGAL

A substance that inhibits the growth of or destroys fungi

ANTIHAEMORRHAGIC

A substance that reduces or stops bleeding when taken internally

ANTIHYPERHIDROTIC

A substance that reduces excessive sweating

ANTI-INFLAMMATORY

See also Antiallergic, Antirheumatic, Antiedematous, Immune depressant)

A substance that reduces inflammation

ANTILITHIC

A substance that reduces the formation of calculi (stones) in the urinary tract

ANTIMICROBIAL

See also Antibacterial, Antifungal, Antiparasitic, Antiviral, Antiprotozoal

A substance that inhibits the growth of or destroys micro-organisms

ANTIOBESITY

A substance that assists in the reduction of body weight

ANTIOEDEMATOUS

A substance that prevents or alleviates oedema (fluid retention)

ANTIOXIDANT

A substance that protects against oxidation and free radical damage

ANTI-PAF

A substance that inhibits the activity of platelet activating factor (PAF). (PAF is a potent inflammatory agent and inducer of systemic anaphylactic symptoms)

ANTIPARASITIC

A substance that inhibits the activity of or kills parasites, especially protozoa

ANTIPLATELET

A substance that reduces platelet aggregation (and hence prolongs bleeding time and may prevent thrombus formation)

ANTIPROSTATIC

A substance that reduces symptoms from the prostate gland

ANTIPROTOZOAL

A substance that kills protozoa or inhibits their growth and activity

ANTIPRURITIC

A substance that relieves or prevents itching

ANTIPSORIATIC

A substance that tends to relieve the symptoms of psoriasis

ANTIPYRETIC

A substance that reduces or prevents fever

ANTIRHEUMATIC

A substance that prevents or relieves rheumatic symptoms

ANTISEPTIC

See Antimicrobial

ANTISPASMODIC

See Spasmolytic

ANTITHYROID

A substance that reduces the activity of the thyroid gland

ANTITUMOUR

A substance that has activity against a malignant tumour

ANTITUSSIVE

A substance that reduces the amount or severity of coughing

ANTIULCER

A substance that prevents or relieves ulceration (usually in the gastrointestinal tract)

ANTIURAEMIC

A substance that reduces the levels of urea in the blood (especially in kidney failure)

ANTIVIRAL

A substance that inhibits the growth of or destroys viruses

ANXIOLYTIC

A substance that alleviates anxiety

APERIENT

See Cathartic

APHRODISIAC

A substance that stimulates sexual desire or libido

AROMATIC DIGESTIVE

A substance that is generally pleasant tasting and/or smelling that assists digestion. They are warming to the body and are also known as warming digestive tonics

ASTRINGENT

A substance that causes constriction of mucous membranes and exposed tissues, usually by precipitating proteins. This has the effect of producing a barrier on the mucus or exposed surfaces

BITTER TONIC

Also known as a Bitter
See also Gastric stimulant

A substance that is bitter tasting and stimulates the upper gastrointestinal tract via the bitter-sensitive taste buds of the mouth and/or by direct interaction with gastrointestinal tissue. Bitters have a promoting effect on all components of upper digestive function, namely the stomach, liver and pancreas. In addition to appetite and digestion they improve general health and immune function

BLADDER TONIC

A substance that improves the tone and function of the bladder and reduces postvoid residual urine

BRONCHOSPASMOLYTIC

A substance that reduces spasm in the lower respiratory tract

CANCER PREVENTATIVE

See also Antitumour

A substance that prevents the incidence of cancer

CARDIOPROTECTIVE

A substance that protects cardiac tissue against hypoxia (oxygen deficiency) and decreases the risk of heart damage

CARDIOTONIC

A substance that improves the force of contraction of the heart

CARMINATIVE

A substance that relieves flatulence and soothes intestinal spasm and pain, usually by relaxing intestinal muscle and sphincters. They are also added to herbal formulations to ease the intestinal spasm or pain that may be caused by laxative herbs

CATHARTIC

A substance that assists or induces evacuation of the bowel and has a strong laxative action. They are also known as purgatives

CHOLAGOGUE

A substance that increases the release of stored bile from the gallbladder

CHOLERETIC

A substance that increases the production of bile by the liver

CIRCULATORY STIMULANT

A substance that improves blood flow through peripheral body tissues. Circulatory stimulants are warming and they support vitality in the body tissues

CNS STIMULANT

A substance that stimulates the central nervous system, increasing alertness

COGNITION ENHANCING

A substance that facilitates learning, memory or concentration

COLLAGEN STABILISING

A substance that stabilises collagen and protects collagen from degradation. Connective tissue tone is thereby improved

COUNTERIRRITANT

A substance that produces a superficial inflammation of the skin in order to relieve a deeper inflammation eg in muscles, joints and ligaments

DEMULCENT

A substance that has a soothing effect on mucous membranes, for example, within the respiratory, digestive and urinary tracts

DEPURATIVE

A substance that improves detoxification and aids elimination to reduce the accumulation of metabolic waste products within the body. They were formerly known as alteratives or blood purifiers and are largely used to treat chronic skin and musculoskeletal disorders

DIAPHORETIC

A substance that controls a fever often by promoting sweating. They are also known as sudorifics

DIURETIC

A substance that increases urinary output

DIURETIC DEPURATIVE

A substance that assists detoxification of the body by the kidneys

DOPAMINERGIC AGONIST

A substance that binds to and activates dopamine receptors

EMETIC

A substance that causes vomiting

EMMENAGOGUE

A substance that initiates and promotes the menstrual flow. Several of these herbs are also regarded as abortifacients

EMOLLIENT

A substance used to soothe, soften or protect skin

EXPECTORANT

A substance that improves the clearing of excess mucus from the lungs by either altering the production and viscosity of mucus or improving the cough reflex

FEBRIFUGE

See Antipyretic

FEMALE TONIC

A substance that improves the tone, vigour and function of the female reproductive system

GALACTAGOGUE

A substance that increases breast milk production

GASTRIC STIMULANT

See also Bitter tonic

A substance that stimulates the function of the stomach

GENERAL BODY TONIC

See Tonic

HAEMOSTATIC

See Styptic

HEALING PROMOTER

A substance that promotes the healing of tissue

HEPATIC (HEPATIC TONIC)

A substance that improves the tone, vigour and function of the liver. This term is vague and other more specific terms are preferable

HEPATOPROTECTIVE

A substance that protects the hepatocytes (liver cells) against toxic damage

HEPATOTROPHO-RESTORATIVE

A substance that restores the integrity of liver tissue

HYPNOTIC

A substance that induces drowsiness and sleep. They are also known as soporifics

HYPOCHOLESTEROLAEMIC

See also Hypolipidaemic

A substance that reduces the level of cholesterol in the blood

HYPOGLYCAEMIC

A substance that reduces the level of glucose in the blood

HYPOLIPIDAEMIC

A substance that reduces the lipid level (cholesterol and triglycerides) of blood

HYPOTENSIVE

See also Peripheral vasodilator

A substance that reduces blood pressure

IMMUNE DEPRESSANT

A substance that reduces immune function and is used particularly where part of the immune system is overactive

IMMUNE ENHANCING

A substance that enhances immune function

IMMUNE MODULATING

A substance that modulates and balances the activity of the immune system

LAXATIVE

A substance that facilitates evacuation of the bowel

LOCAL ANAESTHETIC

A substance that removes sensation or pain when applied locally

LYMPHATIC

A substance that assists detoxification by its effect on lymphatic tissue and often also improves immune function. They are often used when the lymph glands (nodes) are enlarged or tender

MALE TONIC

A substance that improves the tone, vigour and function of the male reproductive system

METABOLIC STIMULANT

A substance that boosts basal metabolic rate

MUCOLYTIC

A substance that helps break up and disperse sticky mucus in the respiratory tract

MUCOPROTECTIVE

A substance that protects the mucous membranes, especially in the context of the gastric lining

MUCOUS MEMBRANE TONIC

A substance that improves the tone, vigour and function of the mucous membranes (particularly of the respiratory tract)

MUCOUS MEMBRANE TROPHORESTORATIVE

A substance that restores the integrity of mucous membranes, eg in the respiratory and digestive tracts

NERVINE TONIC (NERVINE)

A substance that improves the tone, vigour and function of the nervous system. Nervine tonics relax and energise the nervous system

NEUROPROTECTIVE

A substance that helps prevent damage to the brain or spinal cord from ischaemia, stroke, convulsions or trauma

NOOTROPIC

See Cognition enhancing

NUTRIENT

A substance that has a nutritive effect in the body

OREXIGENIC

A substance that stimulates appetite

OESTROGEN MODULATING

In the context of use of herbs, a substance that acts by subtle, poorly-understood mechanisms to promote oestrogen production and/ or effects in the body. The activity may involve interaction with secondary oestrogen receptors such as those in the hypothalamus. They are used to balance hormonal effects, promote fertility and alleviate menopausal symptoms

OVARIAN TONIC

A substance that improves the tone, vigour and function of the ovaries

OXYTOCIC

A substance that causes contraction of the uterine muscle in association with giving birth

PARTURIFACIENT

A substance that induces labour and assists in the efficient delivery of the foetus and placenta

PARTUS PREPARATOR

A substance taken in preparation for labour and childbirth. Treatment usually begins in the second trimester

PERIPHERAL VASODILATOR

A substance that dilates or widens the peripheral blood vessels and thereby improves circulation to peripheral tissues and may assist in reducing blood pressure

PROGESTEROGENIC

A substance that promotes the effect or production of progesterone

PROLACTIN INHIBITOR

A substance that inhibits the secretion of prolactin

PUNGENT

A hot-tasting substance that acts upon a common group of nerve cell receptors having the effect of warming the body and improving digestion and circulation

PURGATIVE

See Cathartic

REFRIGERANT

A substance that has cooling properties, particularly when applied to the skin

RUBEFACIENT

See Counterirritant

Rubefacients are mild counterirritants

SEDATIVE (MILD)

A substance that reduces activity, particularly in the nervous system and decreases nervous tension. It may alleviate pain, anxiety or spasm and induce sleep

SEXUAL TONIC

A substance that improves the tone, vigour and function of the sexual organs

SIALAGOGUE

A substance that increases the secretion of the salivary glands

SKELETAL MUSCLE RELAXANT

A substance that relaxes skeletal muscle tone

SPASMOLYTIC

A substance that reduces or relieves smooth muscle spasm (involuntary contractions)

STIMULANT

A substance that heightens the function of an organ or system eg a central nervous stimulant increases the activity of the central nervous system, particularly behavioural alertness, agitation, or excitation. The term has a second, more subtle meaning derived from the Thomsonian system (an early branch of herbal therapy in the USA): a substance capable of increasing the action or energy of the living body

STYPTIC

A substance that stops bleeding when applied locally

THYMOLEPTIC

See also Antidepressant

A substance that elevates mood

THYROID STIMULANT

A substance that enhances the activity of the thyroid gland

TISSUE PERFUSION ENHANCING

A substance that enhances the flow of nutrients into a tissue

TONIC

Also known as General body tonic
See also other specific body tonics

A substance that improves the tone, vigour and function of the whole body. Tonics can give a boost in energy

TROPHORESTORATIVE

A substance that has a healing and restorative action on a specific organ or tissue

TSH ANTAGONIST

A substance that blocks the activity of TSH (thyroid stimulating hormone)

URINARY ANTISEPTIC

A substance that inhibits the growth of or destroys microorganisms within the urinary tract

URINARY DEMULCENT

A substance that has a soothing effect on mucous membranes of the urinary tract

UTERINE ANTIHAEMORRHAGIC

A substance that reduces the menstrual flow when taken internally

UTERINE SEDATIVE

A substance that reduces the activity of the uterine muscle

UTERINE TONIC

A substance that increases the tone of the uterine muscle

VASOCONSTRICTOR

A substance that constricts or narrows the blood vessels

VASODILATOR

A substance that dilates or widens the blood vessels

VASOPROTECTIVE

A substance that protects the integrity of the blood vessels, especially the fine and more delicate ones

VENOTONIC

A substance that improves the tone and function of the veins

VERMIFUGE

See Anthelmintic

VULNERARY

See also Antiulcer, Astringent, Demulcent

A substance that promotes the healing of wounds when applied locally

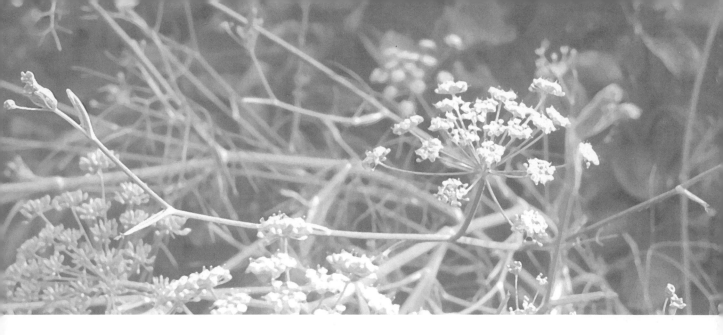

Example Tablet & Capsule Formulations

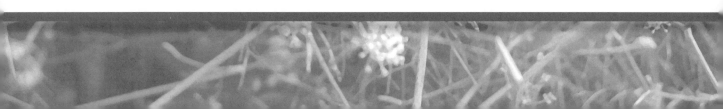

ALLERGY SUPPORT

Albizia lebbeck (Albizia) extract equivalent to dry bark	800 mg
Scutellaria baicalensis (Baical Skullcap) extract equivalent to dry root	800 mg
Tanacetum parthenium (Feverfew) extract equivalent to dry herb	50 mg

ANXIETY SUPPORT

Piper methysticum (Kava) aqueous extract equivalent to dry root containing kava lactones 50 mg	3.2 g

AUTOIMMUNE FORMULA

Rehmannia glutinosa (Rehmannia) extract equivalent to dry root	350 mg
Bupleurum falcatum (Bupleurum) extract equivalent to dry root	700 mg
Hemidesmus indicus (Hemidesmus) extract equivalent to dry root	500 mg
Tanacetum parthenium (Feverfew) extract equivalent to dry herb	165 mg

BILBERRY

Vaccinium myrtillus (Bilberry) extract equivalent to fresh fruit standardised to contain anthocyanosides 15 mg	6.0 g

BOSWELLIA COMBINATION

Boswellia serrata (Boswellia) extract equivalent to dry gum oleoresin standardised to contain boswellic acids 180 mg	1.2 g
Curcuma longa (Turmeric) extract equivalent to dry rhizome standardised to contain curcuminoids 70.4 mg	2.0 g
Apium graveolens (Celery) extract equivalent to dry fruit	1.0 g
Zingiber officinale (Ginger) extract equivalent to dry rhizome	300 mg

BOWEL FLORA COMPLEX

Andrographis paniculata (Andrographis) extract equivalent to dry herb containing andrographolide 10 mg	1.0 g
Tabebuia avellanedae (Pau d'Arco) extract equivalent to dry stem bark	500 mg
Anise (Pimpinella anisum) fruit essential oil	125 mg
Oregano (Origanum vulgare) herb essential oil	75 mg

CAT'S CLAW IMMUNE FORMULA

Uncaria tomentosa (Cat's Claw) extract equivalent to dry inner stem bark	1.5 g
Tabebuia avellanedae (Pau d'Arco) extract equivalent to dry inner stem bark	500 mg
Echinacea purpurea (Echinacea) extract equivalent to dry root	500 mg

CHASTE TREE

Vitex agnus-castus (Chaste Tree) extract equivalent to dry fruit — 500 mg

CHRONIC LUNG SUPPORT

Curcuma longa (Turmeric) extract equivalent to dry rhizome standardised to contain curcuminoids 38 mg — 1.0 g

Ginkgo biloba (Ginkgo) extract equivalent to dry leaf standardised to contain ginkgo flavone glycosides 4.8 mg — 1.0 g

Adhatoda vasica (Adhatoda) extract equivalent to dry leaf — 750 mg

Scutellaria baicalensis (Baical Skullcap) extract equivalent to dry root — 500 mg

Grindelia camporum (Grindelia) extract equivalent to dry herb — 300 mg

Foeniculum vulgare (Fennel) fruit/seed essential oil — 5 mg

CLEAR LUNG FORMULA

Glycyrrhiza glabra (Licorice) extract equivalent to dry root — 500 mg

Verbascum thapsus (Mullein) extract equivalent to dry leaf — 470 mg

Grindelia camporum (Grindelia) extract equivalent to dry herb — 280 mg

Euphorbia hirta (Euphorbia) extract equivalent to dry herb — 280 mg

Zingiber officinale (Ginger) extract equivalent to dry rhizome — 180 mg

Thymus vulgaris (Thyme) herb flowering essential oil — 12 mg

Foeniculum vulgare (Fennel) fruit/seed essential oil — 12 mg

COLEUS FORSKOHLII

Coleus forskohlii (Coleus) extract equivalent to dry root standardised to contain forskolin 18.7 mg — 3.74 g

DONG QUAI

Angelica polymorpha (A. sinensis, Dong Quai) extract equivalent to dry root — 1.0 g

ECHINACEA FORMULA

Echinacea angustifolia (Echinacea) extract equivalent to dry root containing alkylamides 2.5 mg — 600 mg

Echinacea purpurea (Echinacea) extract equivalent to dry root containing alkylamides 2.5 mg — 675 mg

EVENING PRIMROSE OIL CAPSULE

Oenothera biennis (Evening Primrose) seed oil standardised to contain gamma-linolenic acid (GLA) 100 mg — 1.0 g

Appendix 2: Example Tablet & Capsule Formulations

GASTRIC MUCOSAL SUPPORT

Glycyrrhiza glabra (Licorice) extract equivalent to dry root containing glycyrrhizinic acid not more than 1%	3.42 g
Matricaria recutita (Chamomile) extract equivalent to dry flower	600 mg
Filipendula ulmaria (Meadowsweet) extract equivalent to dry herb	500 mg
Matricaria recutita (Chamomile) flower essential oil	5 mg

GINKGO

Ginkgo biloba (Ginkgo) extract equivalent to dry leaf standardised to contain ginkgo flavone glycosides 9.6 mg standardised to contain ginkgolides & bilobalide 2.4 mg	2.0 g

GLUCOSE METABOLISM SUPPORT

Gymnema sylvestre (Gymnema) extract equivalent to dry leaf standardised to contain gymnemic acids 100 mg	4.0 g

GOLDEN SEAL

Hydrastis canadensis (Golden Seal) extract equivalent to dry root & rhizome	500 mg

HAWTHORN

Crataegus monogyna (Hawthorn) extract equivalent to dry herb flowering top standardised to contain vitexin-2-rhamnoside 6.68 mg standardised to contain catechin polymers 15 mg	1.0 g

HERBAL ANTIOXIDANT

Vitis vinifera (Grape) extract equivalent to dry seed standardised to contain procyanidins 42.5 mg	6.0 g
Curcuma longa (Turmeric) extract equivalent to dry rhizome standardised to contain curcuminoids 70.4 mg	2.0 g
Camellia sinensis (Green Tea) extract equivalent to dry leaf standardised to contain catechins 83.35 mg	1.0 g
Rosmarinus officinalis (Rosemary) extract equivalent to dry leaf	1.0 g

HERBAL BOWEL SUPPORT

Rhamnus purshianus (Cascara) extract equivalent to dry stem bark	560 mg
Taraxacum officinale (Dandelion) extract equivalent to dry root	375 mg
Rumex crispus (Yellow Dock) extract equivalent to dry root	375 mg
Anethum graveolens (Dill) extract equivalent to dry seed	375 mg
Matricaria recutita (Chamomile) extract equivalent to dry flower	280 mg

HERBAL THYROID SUPPORT (LARGE SIZE)

Fucus vesiculosus (Bladderwrack) extract equivalent to dry herb containing iodine 600 mcg	1.05 g
Bacopa monnieri (Bacopa) extract equivalent to dry herb standardised to contain bacosides calculated as bacoside A 25 mg	2.5 g
Withania somnifera (Withania) extract equivalent to dry root	600 mg

HERBAL THYROID SUPPORT (SMALL SIZE)

Fucus vesiculosus (Bladderwrack) extract equivalent to dry herb containing iodine 250 mcg	437.5 mg
Bacopa monnieri (Bacopa) extract equivalent to dry herb standardised to contain bacosides calculated as bacoside A 10 mg	1.0 g
Withania somnifera (Withania) extract equivalent to dry root	250 mg

HIGH ALLICIN RELEASING GARLIC

Allium sativum (Garlic) extract equivalent to bulb containing alliin 4.3 mg	1.04 g
Allium sativum (Garlic) dry bulb powder containing alliin 1.4 mg	100 mg

HIGH POTENCY TRIBULUS LEAF

Tribulus terrestris (Tribulus) extract equivalent to dry herb (aerial parts) standardised to contain a minimum of furostanol saponins as protodioscin 100 mg	2.83 g

HIGH POTENCY WILLOW BARK TABLET

Salix purpurea (Willow) extract equivalent to dry stem bark standardised to contain salicin 60 mg	8.0 g

LIVER DETOX ASSIST

Silybum marianum (St Mary's Thistle) extract equivalent to dry fruit standardised to contain flavanolignans calculated as silybin 24 mg	2.1 g
Schizandra chinensis (Schisandra) extract equivalent to dry fruit	1.0 g
Rosmarinus officinalis (Rosemary) extract equivalent to dry leaf	500 mg

LIVER PROTECTION FORMULA

Silybum marianum (St Mary's Thistle) extract equivalent to dry fruit standardised to contain flavanolignans calculated as silybin 168 mg	14.7 g

LIVER/BILIARY TONIC

Silybum marianum (St Mary's Thistle) extract equivalent to dry fruit standardised to contain flavanolignans calculated as silybin 80 mg	7.0 g
Cynara scolymus (Globe Artichoke) extract equivalent to dry leaf	800 mg
Taraxacum officinale (Dandelion) extract equivalent to dry root	400 mg
Bupleurum falcatum (Bupleurum) extract equivalent to dry root	300 mg
Chionanthus virginica (Fringe Tree) extract equivalent to dry root bark	160 mg

LONG TERM IMMUNE SUPPORT

Astragalus membranaceus (Astragalus) extract equivalent to dry root	850 mg
Eleutherococcus senticosus (Siberian Ginseng) extract equivalent to dry root standardised to contain eleutheroside E 600 mcg	750 mg
Echinacea purpurea (Echinacea) extract equivalent to dry root	650 mg

MEMORY/BRAIN TONIC

Bacopa monnieri (Bacopa) extract equivalent to dry herb standardised to contain bacosides 37.5 mg	3.75 g
Schizandra chinensis (Schisandra) extract equivalent to dry fruit	660 mg
Eleutherococcus senticosus (Siberian Ginseng) extract equivalent to dry root standardised to contain eleutheroside E 400 mcg	500 mg
Rosmarinus officinalis (Rosemary) herb top flowering essential oil	10 mg

MENOPAUSE SUPPORT

Dioscorea villosa (Wild Yam) extract equivalent to dry root & rhizome	400 mg
Asparagus racemosus (Shatavari) extract equivalent to dry root	400 mg
Cimicifuga racemosa (Black Cohosh) extract equivalent to dry root	100 mg
Hypericum perforatum (St John's Wort) extract equivalent to dry herb flowering top containing hypericin 333 mcg	600 mg
Salvia officinalis (Sage) extract equivalent to dry herb	290 mg
Panax ginseng (Korean Ginseng) extract equivalent to dry root standardised to contain ginsenosides calculated as Rg_1 & Rb_1 1.4 mg	75 mg

MUSHROOM IMMUNE FORMULA

Ganoderma lucidum (Reishi) extract equivalent to dry mushroom	6.6 g
Lentinula edodes (Shiitake) extract equivalent to dry mushroom	800 mg

NERVOUS SYSTEM TONIC

Hypericum perforatum (St John's Wort) extract equivalent to dry herb flowering top standardised to contain hypericin 413 mcg	750 mg
Schizandra chinensis (Schisandra) extract equivalent to dry fruit	675 mg
Turnera diffusa (Damiana) extract equivalent to dry leaf	625 mg
Scutellaria lateriflora (Skullcap) extract equivalent to dry herb	500 mg

PROSTATE SUPPORT

Serenoa serrulata (Saw Palmetto) liposterolic extract equivalent to dry fruit containing Serenoa serrulata fatty acids 101 mg	1.07 g
Crateva nurvala (Crataeva) extract equivalent to dry bark	900 mg
Urtica dioica (Nettle Root) extract equivalent to dry root	666 mg

SHEEP SORREL FORMULA

Arctium lappa (Burdock) dry root powder	242 mg
Rumex acetosella (Sheep Sorrel) dry herb powder	130 mg
Ulmus rubra (Slippery Elm) dry stem bark powder	32 mg
Rheum palmatum (Rhubarb) dry root powder	8 mg

SHORT TERM IMMUNE SUPPORT

Andrographis paniculata (Andrographis) extract equivalent to dry leaf standardised to contain andrographolide 50 mg	2.0 g
Ocimum tenuiflorum (Holy Basil) extract equivalent to dry herb	500 mg
Echinacea purpurea (Echinacea) extract equivalent to dry root	300 mg
Echinacea angustifolia (Echinacea) extract equivalent to dry root	200 mg
Ocimum tenuiflorum (Holy Basil) leaf essential oil	10 mg

SHORT TERM LOWER RESPIRATORY SUPPORT

Glycyrrhiza glabra (Licorice) extract equivalent to dry root	750 mg
Asclepias tuberosa (Pleurisy Root) extract equivalent to dry root	375 mg
Echinacea purpurea (Echinacea) extract equivalent to dry root	375 mg
Marrubium vulgare (White Horehound) extract equivalent to dry herb	180 mg
Zingiber officinale (Ginger) extract equivalent to dry rhizome	180 mg
Thymus vulgaris (Thyme) herb flowering essential oil	10 mg

SKIN/ELIMINATION SUPPORT

Galium aparine (Clivers) extract equivalent to dry herb	360 mg
Smilax ornata (Sarsaparilla) extract equivalent to dry root & rhizome	360 mg
Berberis aquifolium (Oregon Grape) extract equivalent to dry root & rhizome	360 mg
Arctium lappa (Burdock) extract equivalent to dry root	270 mg
Rumex crispus (Yellow Dock) extract equivalent to dry root	270 mg

SLEEP SUPPORT

Valeriana edulis (Mexican Valerian) equivalent to dry root & rhizome	1.0 g

SLEEP/ANXIETY SUPPORT

Valeriana officinalis (Valerian) extract equivalent to dry root & rhizome	700 mg
Passiflora incarnata (Passionflower) extract equivalent to dry herb	500 mg
Zizyphus spinosa (Zizyphus) extract equivalent to dry seed	900 mg

SLIPPERY ELM

Ulmus rubra (Slippery Elm) stem bark powder	400 mg

SMOOTH MUSCLE RELAXANT

Corydalis ambigua (Corydalis) extract equivalent to dry tuber	600 mg
Zingiber officinale (Ginger) extract equivalent to dry rhizome	400 mg
Rubus idaeus (Raspberry) extract equivalent to dry leaf	400 mg
Dioscorea villosa (Wild Yam) extract equivalent to dry root & rhizome	400 mg
Viburnum opulus (Cramp Bark) extract equivalent to dry stem bark	400 mg

ST JOHN'S WORT

Hypericum perforatum (St John's Wort) extract equivalent to dry herb flowering top standardised to contain hypericin 990 mcg standardised to contain flavonoid glycosides 18 mg	1.8 g

STRESS ADAPT

Eleutherococcus senticosus (Siberian Ginseng) extract equivalent to dry root standardised to contain eleutheroside E 950 mcg	1.25 g

STRESS CONTROL

Withania somnifera (Withania) extract equivalent to dry root	950 mg
Glycyrrhiza glabra (Licorice) extract equivalent to dry root	750 mg
Scutellaria lateriflora (Skullcap) extract equivalent to dry herb	470 mg
Panax ginseng (Korean Ginseng) extract equivalent to dry root standardised to contain ginsenosides calculated as Rg_1 & Rb_1 1.86 mg	100 mg

UPPER DIGESTIVE FORMULA

Silybum marianum (St Mary's Thistle) extract equivalent to dry fruit	2.1 g
Taraxacum officinale (Dandelion) extract equivalent to dry root	500 mg
Citrus reticulata (Chen Pi) extract equivalent to dry fruit peel	500 mg
Gentiana lutea (Gentian) extract equivalent to dry root	100 mg
Zingiber officinale (Ginger) extract equivalent to dry rhizome	100 mg
Citrus reticulata (Mandarin) fruit peel essential oil (cold pressed)	12.5 mg
Matricaria recutita (Chamomile) flower essential oil	5 mg

The coating of this tablet should contain a quantity of Gentian to provide a bitter taste as swallowed

UPPER RESPIRATORY TRACT SUPPORT

Euphrasia officinalis (Eyebright) extract equivalent to dry herb	650 mg
Solidago virgaurea (Golden Rod) extract equivalent to dry herb	650 mg
Echinacea purpurea (Echinacea) extract equivalent to dry root	370 mg
Hydrastis canadensis (Golden Seal) extract equivalent to dry root and rhizome	125 mg
Capsicum annuum (Cayenne) extract equivalent to dry fruit	10 mg

URINARY TRACT SUPPORT

Vaccinium macrocarpon (Cranberry) juice concentrate equivalent to fresh fruit	2.5 g
Crateva nurvala (Crataeva) extract equivalent to dry stem bark	1.0 g
Arctostaphylos uva-ursi (Bearberry) extract equivalent to dry leaf	500 mg
Barosma betulina (Buchu) leaf essential oil	12 mg

VEIN FORMULA

Aesculus hippocastanum (Horsechestnut) extract equivalent to dry seed standardised to contain escin 40 mg	1.2 g
Ruscus aculeatus (Butcher's Broom) extract equivalent to dry root & rhizome standardised to contain ruscogenin 20 mg	800 mg
Ginkgo biloba (Ginkgo) extract equivalent to dry leaf standardised to contain ginkgo flavone glycosides 7.3 mg	1.5 g

WORMWOOD COMBINATION

Artemisia absinthium (Wormwood) extract equivalent to dry herb	100 mg
Stemona sessilifolia (Stemona) extract equivalent to dry root	1 g
Juglans nigra (Green Hulls of Black Walnut) extract equivalent to dry fruit hull	100 mg
Syzygium aromaticum (Clove) flower bud essential oil	20 mg

Bibliography

Bensky D, Clavey S, Stoger E. **Chinese Herbal Medicine: Materia Medica**, 3rd Edn. Eastland Press, Seattle, 2004

Bone K. **Clinical Applications of Ayurvedic and Chinese Herbs.** Phytotherapy Press, Warwick, 1996

Bone K. **Clinical Guide to Blending Liquid Herbs. Herbal Formulations for the Individual Patient.** Churchill Livingstone, USA, 2003

Bone K. **Articles in Townsend Letter for Doctors and Patients.** 1999 to 2007

British Herbal Medicine Association. **British Herbal Compendium, Volume 1.** BHMA, Bournemouth, 1992

British Herbal Medicine Association. **British Herbal Compendium, Volume 2.** BHMA, Bournemouth, 2006

British Herbal Pharmacopoeia. BHMA, Bournemouth, 1983

Chang HM, But PP. (eds). **Pharmacology and Applications of Chinese Materia Medica.** Volumes 1 & 2. World Scientific, Singapore, 1987

Ellingwood F, Lloyd JU. **American Materia Medica, Therapeutics and Pharmacognosy.** 11th Edn. Naturopathic Medical Series: Botanical Volume 2. First published 1898, reprinted Eclectic Medical Publications, Portland, 1983

Felter HW. **The Eclectic Materia Medica, Pharmacology and Therapeutics.** Naturopathic Medical Series: Botanical Volume 1. First published 1922, reprinted Eclectic Medical Publications, Portland, 1983

Felter HW, Lloyd JU. **King's American Dispensatory.** 18th Edn, 3rd revision, Volumes 1 & 2. First published 1905, reprinted Eclectic Medical Publications, Portland, 1983

Mills S, Bone K. **Principles and Practice of Phytotherapy: Modern Herbal Medicine.** Churchill Livingstone, Edinburgh, 2000

Mills S, Bone K (eds). **The Essential Guide to Herbal Safety.** Churchill Livingstone, USA, 2005

Professional Library, MediHerb Pty Ltd. Available at http://www.mediherb.com.au/?page=literature/index

Trickey R. **Women, Hormones & the Menstrual Cycle. Herbal & Medical Solutions from Adolescence to Menopause.** Allen & Unwin, St Leonards, Australia, 2003